D1050848

Sex, Lies & Triathlon

A hilarious look at the world of triathlon and the colorful characters who compete in it

By Leib Dodell

Published by:

FriesenPress

Suite 300 – 852 Fort Street
Victoria, BC, Canada V8W 1H8

www.friesenpress.com

Distributed to the trade by The Ingram Book Company

For my parents . . . always my biggest fans.

Course Map

Chapter 3 — Training

Chapter 4 — Swim

Chapter 5 — Bike

Chapter 6 — Run

Chapter 7 — Race Day

Chapter 8 — Idiosyncrasies

Chapter 9 — Ironman

Awards Presentation 145

About the Author 147

Introduction

A good introduction is a lot like a good warm-up before a race. It sets the tone. Miss your warm-up, and you're likely to feel uptight and uneasy during the race. But get in a nice easy warm-up and you're likely to relax, enjoy the race and maybe even post your best results.

Or so I've been told. I've been competing in triathlons since 1989, and I don't think I've ever once gotten in a decent warm-up. I'm always much too panicked and discombobulated — racing to get to the start on time, trying to decipher the race organizer's cryptic directions, checking the rear view mirror to make sure my bike hasn't fallen off the rack, and rummaging frantically through my bag to see if I remembered to pack both running shoes.

For people who haven't spent too much time around triathletes, this might seem like surprising behavior. To the uninitiated, triathlon probably looks like serious business. If your only exposure to the sport comes from seeing the Hawaii Ironman on TV, or watching that frighteningly intense colleague down the hall who runs to work in the rain and whose office always smells like chlorine, it's easy to see how you could come to the conclusion that your average triathlete is some kind of obsessive, hyper-competitive, anal-retentive, narcissistic freak.

Well, I'm hopeful that the stories and anecdotes in this book might help persuade the general population that, for the most part, this is absolutely, one hundred percent correct.

Triathletes are a unique breed. Like Jane Goodall with her chimpanzees, I've been living among them for many years now. I've trained with them, raced with them, eaten with them (usually at all-you-can-eat buffets), and gone to their weddings (also often at all-you-can-eat buffets). I think I speak with some authority, therefore, when I say that when it comes to emotional balance, most triathletes' spokes are badly in need of truing, if you know what I mean. For about a decade, I chronicled their often erratic behavior in a monthly column in that well-respected scientific journal, *Inside Triathlon* magazine. After years of procrastinating — a time-honored tradition among triathletes, by the way — I finally got around to collecting the columns in this book.

I've often thought about what first attracted me to the sport of triathlon. I was never a particularly great athlete. I wasn't a star high school swimmer or former elite marathon runner or anything like that. I was a middle-of-the-packer. But as an adult I quickly discovered that, through sacrifice, discipline and simple hard work, I could be just as mediocre at triathlon as I was at every other sport I'd attempted.

But the rewards were so much greater. I'm not talking about "personal satisfaction" or "sense of accomplishment" or anything like that. I'm talking pure image here. It didn't matter that I wasn't particularly good at it. The mere fact that I was a *triathlete* got people to oooh and aaah. It was like I had sailed around the world in a balloon or something. Tell someone you sailed around the world in a balloon, and they aren't going to ask you if you broke 19 days. They're just going to walk away shaking their head and muttering, "Man, that dude sailed around the world in a balloon!" You don't get that reaction from tennis, let me tell you, I don't care how nasty your backhand is.

It's a little different now, of course. The mystique has faded a bit. Triathlon has become much more a part of our popular culture. You can get triathlon ties, you can pick up triathlon wrapping paper at CVS for heaven's sake. Instead of being the lone triathlete in the family at Thanksgiving dinner, now you're just as likely to find out that your favorite aunt is recovering from her first half Ironman. And she beat your best time by a good fifteen minutes.

But no matter how much the sport evolves over the years, one thing never changes. Triathlon is always going to attract a certain type of person. And that person is always going to try to set up a bike trainer in the aisle of a commercial aircraft so they don't miss a workout during a transcontinental flight. It's in their blood.

A friend once asked me how I managed to come up with comical anecdotes about triathletes every month for ten years. He asked me this with a totally straight face, even though, at that very moment, we had plastic bags rubber-banded over our running shoes, and we were attempting to shovel the snow off one lane of a high school running track so we could get in a regularly scheduled track workout during a snowstorm. "Um . . . it hasn't been all that tough," I answered, and kept on shoveling.

Chapter 1

Warm-up

You Always Remember Your First Tri

True story: I did my very first triathlon in a pair of old red Converse Chuck Taylors. This was back in 1989. I had absolutely no idea what to expect, and absolutely no idea what I was doing.

This is in stark contrast to the situation today, when I know exactly what to expect, but still have absolutely no idea what I'm doing. I've come a long way.

Like many triathletes, the beginning of my career can be traced back to a basketball game. I was playing in a pick-up game at a local YMCA, landed awkwardly after soaring in for a thunderous dunk (I gotta tell you, it's great being a writer), and suffered a nasty sprained ankle. For the next couple of months, my only hope of getting any exercise was to get the necessary inoculations and jump into the YMCA pool.

It is important to stress here that I had no swimming background of any kind whatsoever. But after a few visits to the pool, analyzing the techniques of the more experienced swimmers, I finally got to the point where I felt comfortable actually putting my face into the water.

After a few weeks of struggling, I was able to swim a couple of laps in a row without stopping and gasping for breath, and I started to delude myself into thinking that I was a "real swimmer." This is a bit like Charlie Sheen thinking he's a Supreme Court Justice — which come to think of it, I'm pretty sure he does at least once or twice a week.

From there, it was only a matter of time before I would enter my first tri. I owned a bike, after all, and I had mastered the basic mechanics of running way back when I was eight or nine years old. Call me a prodigy. So I found a relatively short race listed in a local magazine, and headed down there one Sunday morning with my Raleigh Grand Prix in the back seat of my car.

In retrospect, I was a serious triathlete's worst nightmare. In that one Sunday morning, I think I managed to annoy every single one of the 200-plus competitors at least once. I meandered, Kramer-like, around the transition area, asking extremely idiotic questions of anyone foolish enough to make eye contact with me. I remember thinking that people seemed awfully uptight for what I thought was supposed to be a fun weekend recreational activity.

Then the race started. It was an ocean swim with a beach start that required you to swim straight through the breakers. Within 30 yards, I was treading water, totally disoriented, out of breath and sure I was going to die. I was an instant from turning around, body-surfing back to the beach, and heading home to take up a new hobby. Like Scrabble.

You know how they say that there's a single moment in everyone's life that determines his or her destiny? If I had bagged that race, I probably would've ended up joining a Scrabble club and spending the rest of my life working at an insurance company. Well, I sucked it up and managed to survive that swim. And I still ended up joining a Scrabble club and working at an insurance company. So much for that destiny crap.

Anyway, I remember vividly that I had somehow gotten it into my head that there would be a place to change clothes after the swim. Nevermind that I had spent an hour in the transition area before the start, and there clearly wasn't any such place. I still came out of the water, grabbed my bike clothes, and started wandering around looking for the dressing rooms. I was absolutely shocked to find people getting right onto their bikes and heading out on the course. "You want me to ride my bike in these? But they're *wet!*"

I think about that first triathlon experience every time I go to a race these days. There are almost always a few people at every race who are as clueless as I was at my first event. They're easy to spot — they're the ones wheeling beach cruisers with banana seats into the transition area, or standing at the swim start in Bermuda shorts. As I watch them struggle, I harken back to my first experience and I keep reminding myself — whatever you do, don't make eye contact.

In the Beginning . . .

We like to think of triathlon as a relatively recent concoction, so you might be surprised to discover the Biblical origins of the sport. Consider, for example, this little-known passage: "Ye shall go upon the seas, and take to the titanium horse, and then afoot, lest ye perish . . ." Exodus 140:6.

No wonder the sport is practically a religion to many of us.

Yep, it turns out that triathlon has been around since the beginning of time. (They tried 'em before the beginning of time, but it was really tough to tell who won.) In fact, the first multisport event was actually staged by, of all people, the Jews. This historic race consisted of a short ocean swim, followed by a grueling 40-year march through the desert. Legend has it that sea level was so low the morning of the race that you could practically walk the whole way through. But nobody complained. Imagine the bitching that would go on today.

The course included a brutal climb up the famed Mount Sinai, a climb so intense that competitors were known to hallucinate upon reaching the top. The athletes fueled themselves by eating a high-performance energy food known as "manna," a precursor to the modern energy bar. They rested only to eat, sleep briefly and worship pagan idols.

The race was so grueling that the leader, Moses — a local entrant and crowd favorite (and an inspirational story, since he was competing in the 100 to 120 age group) — actually perished during the run, leaving the race to his protege and training partner, Joshua, who was several thousand cubits back in second place at the time. Moses must've gone out too fast.

Prizes were a heck of a lot better back in those days, too. The promoter of this particular event, for example, promised a Land of Milk and Honey to all finishers, which beats the heck out of an all-cotton T-shirt. This particular prize is still steeped in controversy all these years later. All in all, given the desert sun and all the trouble over the promised Land, everyone probably would've preferred a nice tube of sunscreen.

Tri Finance

Newspapers these days are filled with reports about the Consumer Price Index and the Dow Jones Industrial Average. Instead of talking about sports in subways and over the water cooler, people talk about mortgage interest rates and trends in the stock market. I always feel left out of these discussions, because I have made the economically questionable decision to invest most of my disposable income over the years not in mutual funds or Internet stocks, but in race fees, cycling equipment and the endless other expenses related to the sport of triathlon. Thankfully, I keep virtually no financial records, because it would be truly horrifying to discover just how much money I've dumped into this sport, even though it offers no hope of any financial return whatsoever.

I am sick and tired of opening the paper each morning to read about the latest skyrocketing technology stock that I missed out on. Wouldn't it be nice to open the business section in the morning and see the headline, "Used Shimano components surge 200 percent"? I might not follow the Consumer Price Index, but I can tell you that the Triathlon Price Index seems to be at an all-time high these days. The entry fee for a single race can now run you in the triple digits, particularly if you're foolish enough to register on the day of the race. I think race directors have spent too much time reading tax forms, because race applications nowadays have such a complex set of entry fee calculations that you need to hire an accountant to figure out how much to pay:

- ☐ $80 if you register before May 15 and any other triathlete can claim you as a dependent

- ☐ $95 if you register between May 15 and noon on May 22 and you were born in a leap year

- ☐ $105 if you register after May 22 and you don't want a T-shirt, or you will accept a T-shirt that is so small no adult human being could ever possibly wear it

- ☐ $70 if you are married and racing jointly

Because of the race-day penalty, it always makes good economic sense to register in advance. In fact, you should probably sit down with your financial advisor and map out all the races you're planning to do for the next few years and pre-pay the entry fees. Banks should offer financial tools, like long-term Certificate of Race Deposits (CRDs), to help manage this process, which of course the banks can then collateralize and sell as securities. If you change your mind and decide you don't want to do one of the races, then you should be able to trade racing options the same way investors trade stock options.

Of course, this would require the cooperation of race directors, and good luck with that. Have you ever tried to get your entry fee back from a race director, or even substitute someone else in your place so the money doesn't go to waste? It's tougher than getting the IRS to let you skip a year of income taxes.

The good news is I've finally figured out a solution to our financial woes. Since we've been pouring money into triathlon for so long, I figure it's time to start earning some of it back. So, capitalizing on the popularity of the mutual fund, I've decided to create the Triathlon Fund, a mutual fund that invests exclusively in companies that make all the triathlon-related stuff we end up spending all our money on. Initially, for example, the Tri Fund will invest in Trek, Pearl Izumi, Pam non-stick spray, ziplock bags, pasta, Ben Gay, WD-40, carbon fiber, Velcro, restaurants with All-U-Can-Eat buffets, Vaseline, inner tubes, cheesy motels in beach towns, sunglasses, ibuprofen and bananas. Each month, the Tri Fund will consider new investments based on a detailed analysis of my Visa bill.

If you want to invest in the fund, you'd better get your money in quickly, because it's filling up fast. But you'd better keep track of how much you've invested, because I'm warning you, it's unlikely that I'll have any records.

Tripotenuse

Pythagoras was a mathematician from the 6th century BC who was obsessed with the triangle. Pythagoras's catchy theorem for calculating the hypotenuse of a right triangle — $a^2 + b^2 = c^2$ — is one of the few things most people remember from high school geometry. Using the Pythagorean theorem, if you know the length of any two legs of a right triangle, you can very easily calculate the length of the third leg while at the same time writing out the lyrics to entire Pink Floyd songs on the back cover of your math notebook.

So what does this have to do with triathlon? Well, what doesn't usually make it into the high school textbooks is that Pythagoras was not only obsessed with the triangle, he was also an avid triathlete. In fact, Pythagoras's famous theorem was originally devised to calculate the optimal location to rack your bike within a transition area. If Pythagoras knew the length and width of the transition area, he could calculate the exact rack location that would give him a leg up on all the other 6 century B.C. triathletes. It was centuries before the theory was found to have broader applications.

Unfortunately, some of Pythagoras's other triathlon theories never saw the light of day. They were discovered recently by a team of archeologists, along with a 2700-year-old half-eaten PowerBar, which they promptly finished off. For example, one of Pythagoras's lesser-known formulas was the following:

$$s^2 + b^2 + r^2 = C^2$$

This theory treats legs of a triathlon just like the legs of a triangle. Under this theory, every triathlete possesses an innate, immutable level of conditioning (represented by the constant C), which can be calculated at any given point in time by adding the squares of his or her fitness in the swim (s^2), bike (b^2) and run (r^2). The implications of this theory are profound. For example, let's say you spent a ton of time last winter in the pool and on the treadmill, and made huge improvements in your swim and run. This would mean that, mathematically, your conditioning performance on the bike would have to decrease proportionally. This is also known as the Law of Conservation of Fitness. In other words, it is mathematically impossible to achieve peak conditioning in all three legs of a triathlon simultaneously. Although Pythagoras got a lot of abuse from other triathlete mathematicians at the time, who called him a whiner, centuries of empirical evidence suggest that he was exactly correct.

My all-time favorite of the Lost Triathlon Theorems is this one:

$$o = d - (1 + t/a)$$

You know that moment during a race when you feel like you've finally loosened up, when you're in a rhythm and you're ready to crank? I don't know about you, but in my case that moment always seems to come about an instant before the transition area comes into sight, when it really doesn't do me any good. If I'm doing a tri with a 15-mile bike leg and a 5K run, I'll feel tight and miserable on the bike for about 14.5 miles, and then all of sudden I'll start feeling great. . . just in time to toss the bike and put on my running shoes. And then I'll feel like crap for about 3.05 miles, and just as the finish line comes into view, suddenly I'll start feeling like Steve Prefontaine.

I've always chalked this up to general lameness on my part . . . the whole race I'm suffering, and then once my brain realizes there's no more punishment I can inflict on myself, all of a sudden it starts telling me I feel great and I should crank it up. But Pythagoras proved it mathematically. Under his theory, the optimum moment during any leg of a race (o) is mathematically bound to occur at the distance of that leg (d) minus one instant before the sight of the transition area (1 + t/a).

There are many more great tri theorems to pass along, but I'm also mindful of one of the fundamental mathematical theories of writing: sw = btd-1. In layman's terms, stop writing (sw) at least one word before the reader gets bored to death (btd). Hopefully I'm not too late; I never was much good at math.

Energy Bar Hopping

The issue of nutrition has been eating away at me lately. Nutrition used to be relatively simple. When we were kids, all you had to remember was the "food pyramid," a very user-friendly chart which instructed you to eat several portions of each major food group, represented on the chart by easily identifiable symbols, like a miniaturized cow for "meat" and a stack of hay for "grains." Anyone could understand this, even a kid like me, whose one major food group at the time could be represented by another easily identifiable symbol, namely, the Golden Arches.

Now, however, things have gotten ridiculously complex. We have gone from a straightforward food pyramid to more of a four-dimensional food dodecahedron. The other day, for example, I was speaking about nutrition with a triathlete, always a mistake to begin with, and she told me that blueberries are critical to a healthy diet because they are rich in antioxidants, which help neutralize the free radicals in my blood. Either that, or because they are rich in free radicals, which help neutralize the antioxidants. I can't remember which, because prior to that moment I had thought Free Radicals was a rock band.

One of the big problems with nutrition is that they keep changing the rules on us. Just when you think you've gotten some basic principles down, like "carbohydrates good, fat bad," out comes a new study that says "carbohydrates bad, protein good." You really have to take these nutrition studies with a grain of salt. The reports almost always start out something like this: "If you haven't heard of PHLOGISTON, then you might be interested to know that researchers have discovered that this adenoidal sulfate is the key to unlocking peak performance in endurance athletes!" And then, of course, it turns out that the study just happened to be commissioned by the manufacturers of — surprise! — PHLOGISTON-PX, the new dietary supplement.

I have an additional handicap when it comes to nutrition, which is that my knowledge of the subject is so remedial that even if I could identify the particular nutrients that I was supposed to eat a lot of, I wouldn't really have any idea what foods I could find them in. I have caught on to the idea that there are apparently a ton of carbohydrates in pasta, but beyond that I'm lost. It's not like you can go to the supermarket and ask the guy behind the deli counter where the glycogen aisle is.

Those health food stores don't help the situation much either. They're always staffed by some kid who looks so souped up on chemicals that he might explode at any moment. I wandered into one of these places recently, naively looking for a simple little bottle of multivitamins to help supplement my diet. Not a chance. The walls of these places are lined with jar after jar of increasingly bizarre products with incredibly specific applications. They have supplements that you take before your workout, during your workout, after your workout, when you're thinking about working out, when you have no intention of working out. . . It's totally out of control. If only they'd invent one that you could take *instead* of your workout.

Regardless of which jar you buy, each of them is filled with an identical looking whitish powder that looks like plain old flour to me, and each one goes for about $179.95, with your discount card. If you take it as directed, which is about two shovelsful per glass of water, it will last you about three days. Not a bad business, if you ask me.

The people who have really cashed in on the current nutrition obsession are, ironically enough, the junk food manufacturers, who have discovered the awesome marketing power of the "energy bar." The basic principle here is that if you put a food product in a snazzy wrapper, give it a high-tech name with the words "energy" or "health" in there somewhere, and charge six times as much as a Milky Way, the American consumer will buy them by the boxload, even though they taste like the tongues from old running shoes, which they just might be. Just about every food company on the planet is starting to realize they'd better get on the energy bar bandwagon before it's too late. I understand that Hostess has started crushing the Twinkie into dense, practically inedible patties, and marketing them as high-energy "Twink Bars." It is only a matter of time before Jell-O comes out with its own high energy product — named, of course, "Power Jell-O." Now that, I just might eat.

Fool's Gold

OK, can someone explain to me why there's been Olympic distance triathlons long before triathlon was an Olympic sport? Some of you out there might be too young to remember this, but they didn't have a triathlon in the Olympics until 2000 in Sydney, and I'm pretty sure I was doing Olympic-distance races long before that.

Personally, I'm not so crazy about the idea of triathlon in the Olympics, and I'll tell you why. I remember being totally psyched when I first heard that triathlon was going to be an Olympic sport. "What a great showcase for the sport," I thought. "We'll really put on a show." Months before the race, I started scouring all the tri magazines and racing websites, looking for the "Sydney Olympic Triathlon" entry form. But it was the strangest thing. I found applications for every bizarre race under the sun — the Weasel Breeder's Triathlon, the Prune Festival Triathlon (I hear the lines at the porta-johns move really fast at that one) — but here it was, one of the biggest triathlons ever, and I couldn't even find the darn entry form.

So I started making some phone calls. You think it's tough trying to reach your local race director when you have a question a couple days before a race? Try getting a call back from Juan Antonio Samaranch. I even sent a SASE to the International Olympic Committee. Nothing.

I already had my ticket to Sydney, so I packed up my gear and headed there anyway. I figured I'd just get there early and do race-day registration — it would be a pain in the butt and probably cost a little more, but heck, this is the Olympics. I arrived the day before the race, and I remember thinking, "Boy, triathlon sure is a bigger deal here in Australia than it is in the States." There was a whole lot of excitement about the race, and people seemed really impressed that I was competing. And let me tell you, those Opening Ceremonies beat the heck out of the usual pre-race pasta dinner.

The next morning, I got to the race extra early, to make sure I had time to register and warm up. Things pretty much started going wrong from the beginning. Traffic was a nightmare, and when I finally got there I couldn't find the registration table. And when I tried to wheel my bike into the transition area, suddenly there was quite a commotion. Some of the race officials (it turns out they call them "security" in Australia) came rushing over to grab me, and they were actually quite rude about it.

"What's going on?" I wondered. "Where's the race-day registration table?"

They said I wasn't allowed to race, that only "Olympic" athletes were allowed to compete. I told them there must be some mistake — I'd been racing Olympic distance for years. I could understand having an elite wave, that's cool, but the whole essence of triathlon is that everyone gets to participate, that regular people like me get to rack our bikes and spit in our goggles right next to the fast guys.

The argument didn't go over so well, but at least I got to watch the race from the sidelines, albeit in handcuffs. And I have a couple of observations. First of all, if this was such an important, big-time "Olympic" race, you'd think at least they could do a better job enforcing the drafting rules. One guy in the crowd tried telling me that drafting was actually legal in this race. "Yeah," I scoffed. "And they also allow piggy-back riding during the run." Sometimes spectators can be so misinformed. And then — what a gaffe this was — they made a huge fuss announcing the overall winners, but they completely forgot about the age-groupers!

The bottom line is, for those people who get their first taste of triathlon from watching the Olympics, I'm not so sure they get any real sense of what the sport is really like. I have a suggestion for the Olympic Committee: If you want to see what a real triathlon is like, just stop by any local race on a Sunday morning next summer. Only don't let me spot you — I might have to send some "race officials" over to have a little chat with you.

Will The Real Aliens Please Stand Up

So I'm out for a training ride a couple months ago when all of a sudden these space aliens pull up next to me and ask, "What are you doing?" I wasn't thrilled about being bothered so I replied, kind of snippy, "Why do you ask?" And the aliens explained that they were sent here to find out what Earth people do so they could assimilate into our culture, which sounded like a reasonable explanation to me.

So I told them that I was training for a triathlon, and they flipped furiously through their alien-English dictionaries, but apparently "triathlon" wasn't in there because they gave me a bewildered look and said, "What on Earth is that?" So I explained the sport a little bit, and one of them rolled what I assumed were its eyes and muttered, "And they call *us* aliens," which frankly I took offense at. Another one said that she used to run a little in high school but she doesn't think she could handle the swim. So I told her that's how most of us on Earth feel when we first hear about triathlon, but it turns out the swim isn't that big a deal and you survive it OK. Then she explained that they don't even have liquids on her planet, and I had to acknowledge that this might be a problem.

So the aliens shrug what passes for their shoulders and ask me if there's a decent bike shop around and then zip off, and I didn't think much more about it until a couple weeks later. I'm in the middle of a swim workout, and all of a sudden I can't flip at the wall because there are five new bodies in my lane, which I thought was weird because the rest of the pool was pretty much empty. I was exasperated and I was getting ready to cop an attitude and slip into the next lane when I noticed some-thing strange. The newcomers looked exactly like three Chris McCormacks and two Karen Smyerses, except green and about three feet tall. It was the aliens again. They said hi and asked me if I minded swimming circles.

Turns out the aliens have the ability to assume any human form, and figured they might as well go with the best equipment possible. You can't really blame them for that. The reconfigured aliens asked me what I was doing for a workout, and I told them I was doing a set of 10 hundreds on around 1:30. The aliens gave me this look like I'm from another planet, and then they ducked under the rope and got into the lane next to me. I figured they were worried they couldn't hold my pace, and I'll admit I was feeling a little interplanetary bravado as I pushed off the wall for my next 100, when all of a sudden little green McCormacks and Smyerses started flying by me in the next lane like torpedos. They were doing hundreds on 15 seconds. And that was just their warm-up.

I didn't tell anyone about this — people already have enough doubts about me — and two weeks later I showed up for the first tri of the new season and I noticed even more commotion than usual around the registration table. Sure enough, the alien McCormacks and Smyerses were trying to enter the race, and people were gawking, and it turned out the aliens weren't USA Triathlon members and the race director wouldn't let them register without paying the one-day membership fee, which really pissed the aliens off.

Finally they got this straightened out and everyone was getting ready for the start. The aliens raised some eyebrows by pinning their race numbers directly onto their skin, and one guy who was not *technically* an alien thought this was the newest way to go aero and tried it himself.

Now here's where the story gets a little hard to believe. Turns out that by a bizarre coincidence, the real Chris McCormack and Karen Smyers decided to do this race as a tune-up, and they showed up and registered at the last minute. So the race starts, and the alien McCormacks and Smyerses kick everyone's ass. They average about 300 miles an hour on the bike, they run something like 20-second miles, and they finish the Olympic distance course in a pack in about seven minutes.

As you can imagine, after the race some of the elite non-alien triathletes are not particularly happy about this, and they're telling the race director that the aliens should be in a separate category, since they're a different species, after all, and this certainly shouldn't count in the points rankings, and one guy said he's pretty sure he saw the aliens drafting on the bike.

And I have to admit that I was getting a little bit of satisfaction watching all of this. Because I figured maybe now Chris, Karen and all the other elite triathletes will know how we've been feeling about them all of these years.

Chapter 2

Lifestyle

If Martha Stewart Were A Triathlete...

It's very easy to tell when you're in a triathlete's home. The stacks of old Performance bike catalogues in the bathroom, for example, are a dead giveaway. No matter how hard we try, our places always end up looking like something out of *Better Homes and Derailleurs* magazine.

Our idea of interior decorating is to make sure the colors are properly balanced in the pile of running shoes in the living room corner. If Nike would come out with the Air Feng Shui, it might help us out a little. Yes, it is true that a bicycle can be a work of art. But that doesn't mean hanging muddy commuter bikes from hooks in your living room is a legitimate home decorating technique.

But far and away the most amusing room in the triathlete's household is the kitchen. Every triathlete's kitchen has one drawer that is completely filled with items that were at one time or another in the bottom of a race registration packet — individually wrapped sticks of gum, packets of protein powder, soy pills, salt tablets, half-inch wide PowerBar segments. In the event of a nuclear war, forget about fallout shelters. Just head to the nearest triathlete's kitchen; the food in there is indestructible, and there will be enough to last for years.

The inside of a triathlete's kitchen often bears a close resemblance to the lab at a biotech company. All the "food" is either in powdered form or enclosed in Tupperware. A triathlete's kitchen generally contains more Tupperware than the Grand Opening of a Wal-Mart. This is because triathletes prepare food in large, mess-hall quantities, and are very firm believers in the value of leftovers. A triathlete will never throw food away and will seize every opportunity to hoard it, ant-like, for later consumption.

A recent example will illustrate this phenomenon. A while back, I hosted a group of triathletes who were in town for a local race. One of the younger kids noticed a box of granola bars in my kitchen. He casually asked me if I minded if he tried them, and I said of course not. Then, right before my eyes, he picked up the box, dumped the entire contents into his backpack, said thanks, and walked back into the living room. I swear I am not making that up.

These eccentricities in the areas of dining etiquette and home decorating make for some serious entertainment when a triathlete attempts to host a dinner party. Have you ever been to one of these affairs? You know it's a special occasion when the hosts have chosen to set the table with their very best 20-ounce insulated water bottles. And the dinner napkins have been neatly folded to hide the grease stains from the last time they were used to clean a bike chain. The beverage options consist of water with and without Cytomax.

The good news, however, is that there will be plenty of food. Most triathlete's ideas of group dining come from pre- and post-race buffets, and their dinner parties tend to follow a similar format. There will be large quantities of pasta ladled out of giant tinfoil containers. Bananas will figure prominently in the dessert. Expect long lines, and make sure you attend the pre-dinner meeting.

My Daily Transition

For many years, I worked on the 19th floor of your typical grotesque downtown office building. Because I commuted to work by bike, I left my suits in the office, where they belong. I figured the things are basically uniforms, the lawyer's equivalent of those brown-and-orange McDonald's jumpsuits, except less comfortable. If I worked at McDonald's, as I may well be doing after this book comes out, I certainly wouldn't be wearing my jumpsuit to happy hour, unless of course I had no clean laundry. So why should the business suit be any different?

Anyway, the point is that leaving all my suits in the office had important sociological consequences. The first involves elevators. My daily work routine involved many, many trips up and down the elevators. These trips served the critically important purpose of allowing me to be somewhere other than inside my office, which is where they kept all the work.

What I learned from these trips is that there were only two kinds of people who rode the elevators in my building: business people in suits, and bike messengers in whatever happened to be lying on the floor of the commune that morning. During my first trip up the elevator in the morning, because I hadn't yet changed into lawyer-man, I was indistinguishable from your average bike messenger — as if there were such a thing — except maybe slightly more neurotic. Then, from 9:05 a.m. until (just in case my old boss is reading this) about 6:30 p.m., I turned into your basic annoying business guy in a suit, after which I converted back into a bike dude for the final elevator descent to Earth.

This gave me the unique opportunity to observe the world from both the bike-messenger and business-person perspective, and let me tell you this: When it comes to elevators, Bike People get the shaft.

When I was in the elevator in bike-messenger mode, it seemed like the business-suit people all knew each other. They were always wishing each other good morning and asking about each other's kids or the tax consequences of a withdrawal from their 401(k)s. But they never said good morning to the Bike People. And they would never even consider hitting "DOOR OPEN" for one.

This is not to say that the Bike People were not occasionally shunned for perfectly good reasons, such as because they were standing in the corner of the elevator muttering angrily to no one in particular and furiously scratching their scalps. But the irony is that, psychotics aside, Bike People tend to be far more intelligent than your average lawyer/bureaucrat/weasel in a suit — not surprising, since the bike messengers have figured out a way to ride bikes all day long and get paid for it, while the rest of us are upstairs working our butts off at our computers trying to keep up with our friends' Facebook postings. In fact, most of the time the bike messenger knows the answer to that 401(k) question, but she'll be damned if she'll say anything after the way she's been treated.

You might have picked up on this already, but I always felt like I related much better to the Bike People than the business-suit crowd. Which is why, whenever I'm in the elevator in business-guy mode, I feel like a spy behind enemy lines. I always feel the need to send some kind of coded message to the Bike People, in language only they will understand, that says "I'm one of you." Usually it ends up being something completely lame, like, "So, how do you like those new Shimano SPDs?" As a result, I end up being the only person in the building who is shunned by both the business suits and the Bike People.

It's a Dog's Life

When I was a child, which many people would say is a period of time that has yet to come to a close, we had a dog, Freckles. Freckles' one and only interest, from the moment she woke up in the morning until the moment several minutes later when she took a nap, was consuming as much food as dogly possible. There was no doubt in our minds that, given the opportunity to consume as much as she pleased, Freckles would gorge herself until she exploded like an overinflated inner tube, which is precisely what she came to resemble in her later years.

I have become Freckles. In order to feed my triathlon habit, it seems as though I spend nearly every non-training moment of my life in search of nourishment, like those primitive organisms you read about in biology class. Even when I appear to be doing something completely un-food-related, such as writing this chapter (which doesn't really count, I guess, since it *is* food-related), I am actually thinking intently about the one remaining blueberry-frosted Pop-Tart on the bottom shelf of my kitchen cupboard.

Probably the only significant difference between Freckles and me, food-wise, is that she was a bit more discriminating. She probably would not eat an unwrapped Malt-Nut PowerBar segment found in the back pocket of a cycling jersey after it came out of the dryer. She would sniff it disdainfully, then walk away to suck some lint out of the carpet. I, on the other hand, would scarf it down with the sudden, violent reflex of a frog slurping up a waterbug.

And I don't think I am atypical in terms of general triathlete ravenousness. I base this statement on empirical data collected over years of watching my training partners eat. Have you ever seen a swarm of triathletes descend on an unsuspecting All-U-Can-Eat restaurant after a race or a tough workout? It's not a pretty sight. It's a lot like those nature films of a pack of hyenas devouring a fallen antelope. Except the hyenas have better table manners.

What I can't figure out is why the business community hasn't seized on the well-established link between triathletes and insatiable food consumption with its usual mercenary vigor. The marketing possibilities are endless. Take, for example, those catalogs we get every day, hawking zany cycling jerseys and newfangled bike components. They ought to have special pull-out food sections selling mail-order baked goods and frozen pasta. Entrepreneurial restaurateurs should find out the sites of triathlons in advance and build makeshift take-out shacks right across the street, where they could sell practically any edible food at monopoly prices and make a fortune. And where is Camelbak with the handlebar-mounted, aerodynamic, airplane-like folding tray, so that we can enjoy an in-the-saddle snack on long training rides?

But enough about food for a moment. There is only one activity that can come close to competing with eating on the average triathlete's hierarchy of needs: Sleeping. I am always amused when I read magazine articles telling me that the average person needs only six-and-a-half hours of sleep a night. At least I think that's what they say, because like most sleep-deprived triathletes I usually fall asleep about two or three words into a magazine article.

In my experience, the average triathlete needs about 12 hours of sleep a night, and that's on an easy training week. Few of us manage to get that much, if you don't count work, which can be a lot like sleep, except you're wearing a tie. As a result, we're desperate for bonus pillow time and tend to fall asleep everywhere: at job interviews, on dates, in dentist's chairs. Back when I worked in a big office building, I was tempted on multiple occasions to curl up in a corner of the elevator on the 19-floor trip up to my office to grab a 20-second nap.

Sleep deprivation can be a major burden on our personal lives, which may help explain why so few triathletes actually have personal lives. It rules out, for example, a large number of ordinary social events, like going to a movie. Most triathletes will be out cold before the previews are over. Unless, of course, you keep up a steady stream of Raisinettes.

The Curse of the Common Cold

I think it's fair to say that while triathletes as a group have a number of very positive personal characteristics, common sense is not one that necessary leaps to the top of the list. Many of us have done a couple too many hypoxic workouts, if you know what I mean.

Nowhere is this on display more vividly than in the area of triathletes and the common cold. The average person would probably think that, because of our fanatical obsession with fitness and training, triathletes as a demographic group would rank pretty high on the overall healthiness scale. How ironic, therefore, that according to a recent New England Journal of Medicine report, triathletes as a group now rank, in terms of overall wellness, one notch below Keith Richards. (This type of pop culture reference is always risky, so let me point out that, as far as I am aware, Mr. Richards is still very much alive as of this writing.)

My personal experience is that spending time with triathletes is a lot like hanging out in the waiting room of the local health care clinic, except with more whining. One of the reasons is that the constant training leaves us in a perpetually weakened physical condition. Our immune system is so busy responding to all of the self-inflicted assaults, like those early-morning track workouts in pouring rainstorms, that it has very little left over for all the routine, day-to-day exposures, which makes us sitting ducks for even the most pathetically lame germs that happen to be hovering around out there.

And this is further aggravated by the body-fat factor. Because most triathletes have relatively low body fat, we have very little natural insulation, and we find ourselves bundled up and shivering like a skinny little hairless dog even in the mildest weather. The net result of all this is that in terms of susceptibility to illness, the typical triathlete is pretty much comparable to your average 98-year-old grandmother.

The difference, though, is that the grandmother generally knows what to do when she catches a cold. Triathletes have no clue. I think a lot of triathletes have a tendency to confuse "fitness" and "health." We tend to assume that because we're in generally good physical condition, the normal rules for treating illness don't apply to us. This causes us to do some things that would have given Hippocrates a heart attack. For example, if you have a bad cold and 103 degree temperature, I don't think you will find very many health care professionals who would recommend getting up at 6:00 in the morning to immerse yourself in a freezing cold swimming pool for an hour and a half.

This behavior stems, of course, from the fear that if we ever take a day or two off to rest, we'll get hopelessly out of shape and fall so far behind that our entire racing season, and probably our entire careers, will be trashed. Most triathletes, therefore, won't take time off for any malady short of a severed limb. We've even come up with our own old triathlete's tales to try to justify this behavior. My personal favorite, which I heard just the other day, is that if the cold is in your head, it's OK to train through it; but if it's in your chest, you need to take the day off. I don't believe the Surgeon General has endorsed that one.

As a result, once we do get a cold, there's absolutely no way we can ever get rid of it. It becomes a permanent training partner. I'm pretty sure I've had the same cold for about 14 years now. Although I have to admit there's a pretty good chance that, like a lot of other things, it might literally be in my head.

The Way Triathlon Things Work

They say there's a right way and a wrong way to do things, and if that's true, then I would say I've managed to go through life averaging right about 50-50. And that's my overall average. If you focus only on triathlon-related things, I haven't fared nearly that well.

The problem is that things are just way too complicated. Or at least I like to think that's the problem, because the only other alternative is that I'm way too stupid to figure them out. I think we need a triathlon instruction manual. You might be familiar with the very popular coffee-table book called "The Way Things Work," by David Macaulay, which explains, through the helpful and time-honored pedagogical device of a cartoon elephant, the inner functionings of all kinds of common household items like toasters and toilets.

What we need is a similar book called "The Way Triathlon Things Work," which would demonstrate, with or without the elephant, how all the gear we throw our money at is actually supposed to function. There would be an entire chapter, for example, devoted to the bicycle helmet, or more specifically, the straps on a bicycle helmet. I say "straps," but in fact it occurs to me that I have no idea whether it is actually a series of separate straps or just one single long, extremely tangled strap.

It would be extremely valuable to see a cross-section illustrating what actually happens to the strap(s) once it (they) disappear(s) into the body of the helmet. Because my experience has been that when you tug on one end of a strap, the resistance is felt on another strap in a completely different region of the helmet that seems to bear no logical or spatial relationship to the strap you just tugged on. The result is that it can take weeks of sophisticated computer modeling to figure out exactly which strap needs to be tugged how far in order to produce the desired adjustment.

And then there are those little plastic gizmos on the end of the straps, the ones that snap together to fasten the helmet under your chin. It is a very good thing that the helmet comes with these gizmos already attached to the straps, because once they fall off, you might as well just ditch the whole helmet and head to the bike shop to buy another one. Each of these little gizmos has three small slots on the end, and somehow the strap is supposed to go up through one and down through another and then out through the third in a manner that securely fastens the gizmo to the strap.

I don't know about you, but I have spent hours sitting there staring at the thing and scratching my head, like a chimpanzee in the monkey cage at the zoo, trying to figure out how in the world it's supposed to work. No matter what I do, I always end up either with an unused slot, or with the gizmo pointing in the wrong direction. And when I momentarily think I've gotten it right, the gizmo just slides right off the strap with absolutely no resistance whatsoever, and the only way I can visualize to fix the problem is for the strap to double back right through itself in ways that I'm pretty sure are physically impossible.

"The Way Triathlon Things Work" would walk us through all this, and would take on other equally frustrating devices like the bicycle pump. Bike pump designers seem to have adopted the philosophy that the pump user is in constant telepathic communication with them, so there is no need for the device to contain any actual explanatory information. My floor pump, for example, has a little lever on the end that fastens the nozzle to the valve. I have had this pump for more than a year and I still have no idea whether the lever should be in the down position when you put it on the valve and then lifted up to tighten, or the other way around. My frame pump is even more mysterious. It has two settings: "hp," which for the sake of argument I am willing to assume stands for "high pressure," and "x," and on that one I really can't even venture a guess, although I will say that I am very reluctant to pump a substance known only as "x" into my inner tubes.

"The Way Triathlon Things Work" could also address other important questions like the proper method of placing your bike on the bike rack during a race. I have always been a follower of the traditional front-in, brake-levers-on-the-rack method. But lately I have seen a surge in popularity of the more radical back-in, saddle-on-the-rack method, and I could use some guidance on this. And while we're on the subject of bike racks, I think it would be worth spending a chapter on bike-rack etiquette. How many times have you gotten to a race early, racked your bike and laid out all your gear, only to go out for a little warm-up ride and come back to find some new bike happily racked in your spot?

I recognize that the prelude to a triathlon can be a stressful and chaotic time, but it seems to me that it shouldn't be too difficult to figure out that if there is what appears at first glance to be an open space on a rack, but with a whole bunch of gear laid out on a towel underneath it, there's probably a bike associated with it somewhere. Yet just recently I was at a race and watched with my own eyes (which is how I usually watch) as a friend who had racked her bike next to mine went out for a little warm-up spin. Sure enough, along came an Interloper who cheerfully began to rack in my friend's spot. When I pointed out to the Interloper that the spot was taken, she said OK, and proceeded to walk her bike around to the other side of the rack, and put it in the exact same spot.

I am not sure exactly what her reasoning was. It was true that she was now safely out of harm's way on the other side of the rack, not directly on top of my friend's gear, but it seemed obvious that only one bike could occupy that spot on the rack, regardless of which side it was coming from. A helpful diagram in "The Way Triathlon Things Work" would drive this point home. And I think it would be appropriate to use the diagram to exact a little revenge on the Interlopers of the world — and here is where that cartoon elephant just might come in handy.

No Escaping Alcatraz

Recently, I had a difficult decision to make. Should I leave the East Coast, where I'd lived my whole life, and move all the way across the country to San Francisco to take a new job? It was a tough call, so I did what they always tell you to do in these situations: I made a list of the pros and cons.

At the very top of the cons list, circled three or four times in bright red ink, was one word: Alcatraz. I knew that if I lived in San Francisco and wanted to continue to pretend to be a half-serious triathlete, there would be no way I could escape competing in the famous, and famously insane, *Escape from Alcatraz* triathlon. Fifty-something-degree water, choppy seas, nasty currents, sharks . . . As long as I was safely on the East Coast, I could continue to hide behind the fact that I was 3000 miles away and it was just too far to travel.

It's particularly appropriate that Alcatraz was on my "cons" list because, as everyone knows, Alcatraz was for many years the site of a maximum-security prison for violent felons. In fact, "Pros and Cons" would make a pretty good name for the Alcatraz triathlon, because the only people who seem to have any legitimate business being on the island are professional triathletes and convicted felons.

Alcatraz officials like to boast that no prisoner ever successfully escaped from The Rock. This statistic is a bit misleading. There are actually several prisoners who escaped from their cells and disappeared into the Bay, and who are now listed, officially, as presumed dead. Similarly, Alcatraz triathlon officials like to boast that no one has actually been devoured by sharks during the race. Once again, however, the truth is a bit grayer. There are large numbers of registered competitors who never made it out of the water and who are listed, officially, as presumed to have come to their senses at the last minute and opted for a vanilla soy latte at Starbucks instead.

If there are any living prisoners who did time on Alcatraz, the *Escape from Alcatraz* triathlon must be the ultimate indignity. There they were, the meanest, nastiest, most hardened criminals in the world, afraid to make an escape attempt because they didn't think they could possibly survive the swim. And now, every summer, they have to watch on TV as 2000 yuppies from San

Francisco to New York climb out of their Nissan Xterras, take a ferry to the island and swim back to shore in 45 minutes. It would probably be about the same as we'd feel if, without any training, the Birdman of Alcatraz won the Hawaii Ironman.

To prove beyond doubt that we as a society are spiraling further and further into complete madness, there are now not one but two Alcatraz races every summer, in order to handle the over-flow crowd of triathletes who want to participate. Only the first race, held in June, is the "official" Escape from Alcatraz Triathlon, and it guards that trademark zealously. The second race is held in August, and, after some extensive legal tussling, now has the more generic name of the San Francisco Triathlon at Alcatraz. Maybe they should call this second race Escape from Litigation.

Anyway, despite my list of pros and cons, I did end up moving to San Francisco, and as I feared, I found it impossible to escape Alcatraz. And I even shamed a couple of my old East Coast training buddies to come out and race with me and provide moral support. I did reasonably well — I think I finished just behind the Birdman.

A Healthy Tirade Against Health Clubs

OK, to begin with, I have no idea why they call them "health clubs," because they really don't have much to do with health at all. When is the last time you heard someone at the office yell, "Smithers just passed out in the hallway. Quick! We've got to get him to a health club." Next time you're at your club, try asking one of the trainers for a routine physical, and see what happens.

But "fitness club" isn't much better, because while these clubs have very little to do with health, they might have even less to do with fitness. In my experience the goal of most trendy urban health clubs is to keep their membership hovering somewhere in the range where they aren't so out of shape that they will experience a cardiac event after 90 seconds on the StairMaster, but not in such good shape that they will become an annoyance to other club members or, God forbid, the health club staff.

At my old health club, for example, there was a rule — a giant complex web of rules, actually, but I am thinking of one rule in particular — that members could only use the cardiovascular equipment for 20 minutes during peak hours. "Peak hours" were strictly defined in the Health Club Guidelines as anytime when a person who works a normal schedule and does not happen to be an unemployed drifter is able to go to the health club.

I have a suspicion that the reason for this time limitation was not so much to make sure the equipment was available to all members, but rather because exercise for more than 20 consecutive minutes runs the grave risk of possibly causing the user to sweat, which would not only destroy the aesthetics of the health-club environment, but might also require a member of the health club staff to occasionally clean the equipment and miss valuable time reading *Vogue*, *Shape* and the other highly educational publications behind the Front Desk.

This is an absolutely true story that I swear I am not making up: At my old health club in Connecticut, they had a rule outlawing the wearing of sleeveless shirts in the workout area. If you attempted to mount a treadmill or stationary bike wearing a singlet — keep in mind, this is a garment specifically designed to be worn while running — several grave-faced employees would appear out of nowhere, throw a towel around your naked shoulders, and quickly escort you to the locker room. In a world of inane rules, this one has got to be at the very top of the list. It's a bit like Vail Resort deciding to outlaw ski jackets on the mountain.

You might sense a hint of bitterness in my writing. This may be a result of my experience a while back, when a number of members of a posh, urban health club tried to organize a triathlon team. If you think that the health club staff enthusiastically supported their members' efforts to push their conditioning to the limits by competing in this demanding sport, then you've been sniffing the Tri-Flow again, because this is simply not part of the health club mentality. Instead, it was as if we were a group of kindergartners — OK, I admit there might be a valid analogy there — asking their teacher if they could leave class early to go set fire to the gymnasium.

Suffice it to say, it was a battle every step of the way, from the grave issue of bikes in the pool area — to a health club administrator, bikes in the pool area is the health club equivalent of the Cuban missile crisis — to our failed effort to set up rollers in the aerobics studio. Here's a hint to those of you thinking about starting a triathlon team in your own club: Whatever you do, do NOT mess with the aerobics studio. This is health club Holy Land.

But the mother of all battles was our attempt to reserve pool time for a coached workout. Never mind that we supplied our own coach; that we welcomed — OK, tolerated; OK, didn't try to drown; OK, didn't actually drown — any club members who wanted to join our workout, that no one had ever complained to us personally, and that the pool was generally empty during the hours we wanted to train. Notwithstanding all of this, we were forced to cram into half the pool so that the other half could make itself available to anyone who happened to wander by in search of a refreshing dip. This typically produced the highly comical image of half a pool crammed with 20 thrashing triathletes, while the other half was occupied by a single swimmer with her hair in curlers doing sidestroke in an uncanny impersonation of Esther Williams.

I suspect that this chapter will accomplish little more than reinforcing the average health club member's stereotype of the arrogant, hostile triathlete who hogs the bike paths and the exercise equipment and doesn't give a damn about anyone's workout but his or her own. Then again, maybe not. I think it's unlikely the average health club member will put down *Vogue* or *Shape* long enough to pick up this book.

Tri-ing to Retire

I think we can all agree that one of the easiest things about competing in a triathlon is stopping at the end of the race. All you have to do is get to the finish line, attempt to tear that little tag off the bottom of your race number before giving up and letting the race official do it, and then, well . . . stop. There really isn't much point in continuing to run after that, unless you're in a real big hurry to find a private spot to throw up.

It's ironic, therefore, that outside of an actual race, stopping seems to be one of the hardest concepts for triathletes to comprehend. Stopping, as in retiring, calling it quits, hanging up the wetsuit and racing flats. Admit it, we've all been tempted at one time or another. Some of us have even tried it a couple of times. But very few of us have ever been able to actually get out.

One of the reasons retiring is so difficult for triathletes is that there's no natural stopping point: no Super Bowl, no Final Four, no natural culmination of our career where we can go out in a blaze of glory. For us, there's always another race, another opportunity to shave a couple seconds off our time or move up a couple of spots in the race results.

The age-groupings don't help either, because we convince ourselves that if we can just make it to the next age group, all of a sudden we'll be invincible, there's no way those old geezers will be able to touch us.

But an even more serious obstacle to retiring is that most triathletes have absolutely no idea what to do with themselves once the training and racing disappears. While we're competing, we whine constantly that triathlon leaves no room for all the other important things in our lives. But once we give triathlon up, suddenly we can't figure out what any of those other things are. Training for the next event is what gives structure to our daily lives. We know we've got our running group on Wednesdays, our Masters swim on Tuesdays and Thursdays. Take all these things away, and we're lost.

And then there are the purely physiological aspects of retirement. Over time, our bodies have become accustomed to regular bouts of vigorous, borderline masochistic exercise. This allows us to get away with things that other people's bodies can't even contemplate. How many times, for example, have you been eating lunch in the office cafeteria, a huge pile of pasta and two pieces of pie on your plate, when one of your colleagues says something about how "lucky" you are to be able to eat like that and stay so thin. You want to tell her it isn't so much luck as it is the 8 miles of trail running you put in that morning.

Because retiring poses so many physical and emotional difficulties, most of us just keep on training and racing, year after year, long after it ceases to be exciting or even particularly enjoyable. We're doomed to end up spending our Social Security checks on entry fees and geriatric cycling shorts. Our friends marvel at our dedication, but the reality is that, like addicted smokers, many of us just lack the courage to quit. I have triathlete friends who have attempted to retire more times than Brett Favre. "I'm retired!" they'll declare with total, almost pathetic confidence. Then, a week later, you'll spot them at the track, helplessly running mile repeats.

In my own case, I have to admit that after my second ankle surgery, I thought long and hard about calling it quits. But I guess I'll stick around another couple seasons. If I can just make it to the next age group, there's no way those 50-54-year-olds can beat me.

Chapter 3

Training

Better Late Than Never

OK, so it's April already. You've been goofing around all winter, trying to put the "fun" back into your workouts, doing things like yoga classes and going on "sightseeing" bike tours and (admit it) playing in a volleyball league. And now, all of a sudden, the racing season is approaching fast, and you are not. Is this any reason to panic?

Yes, it most certainly is. If you were planning to start racing in May, you're pretty much screwed. I don't know about you, but it doesn't help reduce my anxiety level to pick up those triathlon magazines filled with article after article describing the kind of training I should have been doing all winter long. You know the articles I'm talking about — the ones that start off with statements like, "Let's say you usually do your one-armed 100 IMs on 55 seconds. This week, to mix things up . . ." When I read stuff like that, it makes me want to toss the author into the deep end of the pool with cement swim fins.

Since the tri magazines have the anxiety-producing-training-tip genre pretty well covered, I thought I would devote this chapter to helpful tips for those training procrastinators out there, those of you who maybe weren't quite as focused as you should've been last winter and suddenly find the racing season staring you in the face.

My first and most critical piece of advice is to forget the idea that you can make up for the lost time just by training especially hard this spring. I know it's a comforting thought. It's basically the exact same theory as "cramming" for exams in college. You didn't touch a textbook from January to May, and then, a day or two before the final, you tried to cram a semester's worth of information into your atrophied brain. And then you probably got an "A" anyway, at least if you went to a state school like I did, which of course just reinforced the idea that you can dig yourself out of any hole.

Well, take my word for it, this one is the Grand Canyon. You will find it far more difficult to cram for a triathlon. You could try pulling an all-nighter on your Computrainer the night before a race, but I doubt it'll help your performance much the next morning. To continue the exam analogy, the next best option that springs to mind is probably cheating. In college you could make it through an art history exam by scribbling the names of Renaissance painters on your forearm, but the only thing that's going to be written on your arm when the first race rolls around this summer is your bib number. I suppose you could try scribbling "GO FASTER" on your palm, just in case you forget the concept, but I don't think it's going to be much help. And don't let the race marshals catch you.

So cramming and cheating are not options, is the point I'm trying to make. But that doesn't mean all is lost. There's another technique that might come in handy, and it's also one we learned back in school. Which makes perfect sense, by the way, since triathlon has basically taken the place of school in many ways in our daily lives. It supplies the same steady doses of stress and feelings of inadequacy, with training taking the place of studying, and race results substituted for report cards. Instead of hoping we get seated next to the hottest girl (or guy) in school, now we hope we get to rack our bikes next to them. When we were in school we had recurring nightmares that we were taking a test, and suddenly realized we weren't wearing any pants. And now, in real life, we compete in triathlons and suddenly realize we're not wearing any pants. The similarities are endless.

But I digress. If you had an exam coming up and you knew there was no way you would be ready for it, what did you do? What you did was try to buy yourself more time by making up some excuse and getting permission to take a make-up exam. Well, the same principle holds here. The basic idea is to push that first race back as late as possible, and use the extra time to catch up on your training. If it's too late to start training early, the next best thing is to start racing late.

Of course, it wasn't easy convincing your teacher that you had a good reason to take that make-up, and it won't be easy convincing your training partners that you've got a good reason to blow off those early season races. I have found that weddings serve really well for this purpose. If you've got an out-of-town wedding the weekend of a big race, people tend to accept that there isn't much you can do about it. They may even sympathize with you, which is an added bonus. So you need to start canvassing friends and relatives to identify weddings on the appropriate weekends, and get yourself invited. I've gotten so good at this, I've had seasons where I didn't do my first race until late September. You shouldn't expect this kind of success your first season, but if you can make it to July or even August, you should be OK.

In Therapy

I hate to be the bearer of bad news, but the truth is that if you keep this crazy triathlon stuff up long enough, sooner or later you're going to have to deal with a serious injury. Clinical studies have proven that, statistically, serious injuries are most likely to occur immediately before the biggest race of your season, and usually while you are engaged in some type of unnecessarily high-risk activity, such as pulling on a sweater.

The likelihood of injury is particularly high if, like me, you insist on continuing to train and race even though you have reached an age when your body has had enough of this type of activity and would, quite frankly, prefer you to take up a pastime that involves less physical wear and tear, such as, for example, chess. Your body has a very clear way of signaling you that this time has come. Your body works a lot like a disgruntled labor union. If it is unhappy with the way things are going, it will suddenly and without warning go on strike and shut down major operations, such as joints and tendons, to force you to take notice and do something about the situation.

In my case, I got a very clear message recently in the form of a torn achilles tendon, which involved surgery followed by an extended period of physical therapy. To continue the union analogy way past its usefulness, physical therapy is the physiological equivalent of the collective bargaining process, in which neither me nor my body is likely to be completely satisfied with the outcome. We are certain to have ongoing conflicts, but hopefully we will be able to reach some type of accommodation that will allow us, grudgingly, to continue operations.

In case you have never gone through the process of physical therapy, I thought it might be helpful to give you some idea of what you can expect. The first thing that you need to know about physical therapists is that, by federal regulation, all physical therapists are required to be drop-dead gorgeous. There is a good public policy reason for this. Health care regulators know that, because of what physical therapists actually do to you, if they weren't preposterously attractive, there is no way anyone would ever consider going to see them in a million years. The job of the physical therapist is to find out what part of your body hurts, and then probe and prod and pull and tug and manipulate and basically inflict as much pain on that particular body part as possible over a sixty-minute period. And then bill your health care provider.

Of course, like most federal regulation, the "drop-dead-gorgeous rule" has the potential to backfire, particularly when applied to triathletes, who are borderline masochists to begin with, and for whom the pain alone would probably be a sufficient narcotic even without the pulchritude. In my case, I typically went to see my physical therapist on Monday-Wednesday-Friday to rehabilitate my Achilles tendon, and then I spent Tuesday and Thursday doing as much as I possibly could to de-habilitate it, so as to the reduce the chance that the therapist would tell me that I'm cured and I don't have to come back. Each time I went back in there, I tried to look genuinely dejected when I announced that it didn't seem like I made that much progress since my last session.

The inside of a physical therapist's office is like a cross between a fitness center and an insane asylum. There are some familiar-looking pieces of exercise equipment, but there are also people engaged in some extremely unfamiliar activities. There are people trying to walk on their hands and knees like a crab with neon-colored elastic bands wrapped around their ankles. There are people lying on their backs attempting to lift giant inflatable balls into the air with their feet. There are people trying to balance themselves on one foot on a wooden board that has been placed on top of a baseball while attempting to play "Flight of the Bumblebee" on a violin.

OK, I made up the part about the violin, but only because the physical therapists haven't yet found the right combination of hallucinogenic drugs to come up with that one. I'm convinced that at the end of the day, after they say goodbye to their last patient and lock the door behind them, the physical therapists turn to each other and say, "You wouldn't believe what I got a guy to do today!"

The Balance Cheat

Finally, after years of struggling to juggle triathlon training with work, family and personal relationships, I am very pleased to announce that I have, at long last, discovered the secret to achieving perfect balance in life. I feel it's my ethical duty as a triathlon journalist to share this with the rest of the triathlon community.

So here you go: The key to achieving perfect balance is to get your life stretched out to the point where you are so overcommitted that you are pretty much equally ineffective at everything you do. In my case, for example, I have tried to back off training just a little bit, and as a result my race results are predictably mediocre. But this is compensated for perfectly by the fact that I train just hard enough to distract me from completely focusing on my job, so my professional results are mediocre as well. And, of course, this is all perfectly balanced by the fact that I spend so much effort scrambling to make time for work and training that my personal life is dissatisfying to boot. What perfect harmony!

Another useful trick to fool yourself into thinking that you have a healthy balance in your life is to focus on increments of time that are long enough to allow things to balance themselves out naturally, based on the law of averages. If you allow yourself to fall into the trap of focusing on days, weeks or even months, of course it's going to seem like you spend an absurdly disproportionate amount of time training for a sport that does nothing for you professionally and has no logical relationship whatsoever to anything else going on in your life.

Try to broaden your frame of reference a bit. Instead of looking at it in terms of days or weeks, try looking instead at, say, your entire life. I'd be willing to bet that for the first 10 or 15 years of your life, you spent very little time training for triathlon. Your last few years are likely to be fairly triathlon-free as well. So even if you've been obsessed with the sport for the last decade or two, in the overall scheme of things you're reasonably well balanced. (Warning: You might find that this argument doesn't go over well with bosses and loved ones. But it is an excellent way to fool yourself.)

There is another type of balance that plays an important role in my life, as I'm sure it does in the lives of most triathletes. The balance I'm talking about here isn't the healthy-lifestyle kind of balance that therapists preach about. It's more the completely psychotic physiological type of balance that only a truly unbalanced triathlete could understand. Example: I generally finish every swim workout with exactly the same cool-down, which includes a set of 50-yard one-arm pulls — left arm, right arm, then left, then right. The other night, I was finishing my workout and racing against the clock because I knew the pool was about to close. Sure enough, suddenly there was a kickboard in my face and the lifeguard kicked me out before the last right-arm lap. I was completely traumatized, because I had done two left arms and only one right, and I was convinced that I was going to be out of alignment for the rest of my life and there was no way I could ever compensate for it. I actually went into the locker room and tried to do some one-armed push-ups in a truly deranged attempt to balance things out.

Latest Training Tip –
The Fundraiser

I have another secret to share, and this time it is nothing less than the triathlete's key to life. I am obviously reluctant to disclose this information to the general public — or even the extremely specific triathlon-book-reading public — so I hope you appreciate the great personal sacrifice I am making here.

The triathlete's key to life is fundraisers.

You know the things I'm talking about — those events where people agree to "sponsor" you by actually donating money for every mile you swim or bike or run. Maybe it's not quite up there with getting sponsored by Nike, but for those of us with no real shot at professional careers — I'm not just talking about professional triathlon careers, I'm talking about any kind of professional career — it's the next best thing.

The beauty of the fundraiser is this: Because it appears to benefit some worthwhile cause, like saving the yak or curing male pattern baldness, it totally legitimizes your training and immunizes you from criticism of any kind. Instead of the usual derisive comments from colleagues and loved ones about self-indulgence and narcissism, people actually thank you and give you free food and T-shirts. It's the ultimate scam. And if a spouse or significant other has the audacity to question your true motivation, you don't have to rely on the usual pathetic justifications for obsessive training, like trying to shave another half second off your 10k time. All you have to do is look 'em square in the eye and say, "This isn't about me. It's about the yaks."

There is so much competition among fundraisers these days that they're constantly adding more and more perks to the deal. There are fundraisers in which they not only feed you and give you a free place to crash for the night, they also tune your bike and do your laundry and prepare your tax returns. Don't these people know I'd still be out here if all I got was half a PowerBar?

If the organizers of these fundraisers really understood the psychopathology of the typical endurance athlete, they'd go about them a bit differently. Instead of asking innocent people to pay for each mile of training, they would be hitting up the athletes themselves, who are training addicts and will make easy targets. If it's a bike-a-thon, ask the triathletes to pledge a dollar for every mile they ride after the first ten. None of them will be able to quit at ten miles. Pattern baldness will be a thing of the past in no time. Better yet, they ought to try a "reverse fundraiser," in which the spouses of triathletes pledge money for every mile their significant others agree *not* to swim, bike or run. They could call it a "non-a-thon" and make a fortune.

The only problem with adopting the fundraiser as a way of life is that it can get tough going back to the same people for money again and again. When people see me coming with one of those pledge forms in my hands, they'll go to extraordinary lengths, including feigning heart attacks, to avoid me. I feel like a process server. It has gotten to the point now where I no longer raise money for specific fund-raising events. I raise money year-round and use it on a revolving basis, like a gant training pyramid scheme. At least you can feel pretty confident that a good chunk of the money you spent on this book will end up going to a worthwhile cause!

The Excuse

In this chapter, I would like to discuss an extremely vital but often overlooked element of your training regimen: The Excuse. Mastering this skill will help you achieve two of the foremost goals of most age-group triathletes: deflecting ridicule, and maintaining an artificially inflated reputation among your training partners and the racing community at large. Remember, you can go fast. . . or you can have a really good excuse for going slow. The excuse hurts less.

Suppose, for example, you meet up with a group after work for a run, and you're really struggling. You're moving slower than the line for the porta-john on race day morning, and the group drops you like a paper cup at a water station. When you finally make it back, the rest of the group has showered, dressed and is afraid to look you in the eye. Do you say: (1) "Sorry guys, I'm weak and lazy and I just couldn't go any faster." Or do you say: (2) "Boy, that century ride this morning really wore me out. Or maybe it was the squats at lunch."

I think you get the picture. Here are a number of useful tips from a veteran that can help make your excuses more effective:

1. Always set up your excuse in advance. You never know which races or workouts are going to reach the excuse threshold, so it's always useful to lay a strong excuse foundation just in case. This may sound difficult, but all it takes is a little "the knees are a bit sore today, but I'll give it a shot," or maybe a quick "that seafood salad I had for lunch feels a little funny" before starting out. Over time, if you put in the necessary repetitions, this will become second nature.

2. Maintain proper form during your excuse. Body language is crucial. Appear angry, frustrated, disgusted. Throw things. Kick your bike. Sulk. You've really got to sell it.

3. Subjective excuses are always better than objective ones. In other words, the less provably false your excuse is, the better. For example, I find — and I know there are experienced fake triathletes out there who

disagree with me on this — that medical conditions, as a rule, are far more effective than equipment failures. It can be very embarrassing to blame a bad ride on, say, a malfunctioning derailleur, only to have some gear-head come by and prove to everyone it's working perfectly. Whereas it would be very unusual for someone to prove your gastrointestinal problems are a sham.

4. You know how they say you should never try a piece of equipment during a race that you haven't tried during training? The same goes for excuses. Make sure your excuses are race-ready. Any slight hesitation or uncertainty can give you away, so proper preparation is essential.

5. Keep an excuse log. Record the type of excuse used, the people to whom it was made, and how it went over. This will avoid overuse problems and guard against the dreaded problem of contradictory excuses — like a tonsillectomy one season and tonsillitis the next — also known as "excuse bonk."

6. There are a couple other things I'd like to share on this topic, but unfortunately I've got to get this chapter wrapped up. I forgot to bring my battery charger and my laptop is about to run out of

This Workout Just Isn't Working Out...

I saw a "Help Wanted" ad the other day for a health club that tried to lure new employees by promising them that they'd "love their work as much as their workout." I got a chuckle out of this. Clearly the creative people who designed this ad are not out there doing hill repeats at 6:00 a.m.

"Love" is not the first word that springs to mind when I think about a workout like that. "Stomach-churning dread" is more like it. But I guess "Dread your work as much as your workout," while maybe higher on the truth-in-advertising scale, doesn't make for the catchiest of slogans. To be fair, though, I really can't say that I completely despise my workouts. It would probably be more accurate to say that I have the classic "love/hate" relationship with them. Basically, a good hard workout to me is like the exact opposite of casual sex: You always dread it beforehand, but afterwards you're always really glad you did it.

The biggest problem with workouts is that, like relationships in general, while they have some very positive overall benefits, they can be extremely stressful to manage on a day-to-day basis. I spend a tremendous amount of mental energy every single day just making sure that nothing goes wrong in my life that will upset that day's workout schedule. And like relationships in general, something almost always goes wrong. For example, if I'm scheduled to do a hard track workout after work one day, odds are extremely high that one of my colleagues is going to plop an enormous leftover hunk of ice cream cake onto my desk at 4:30 that afternoon.

This particular problem, I must admit, is partly my own doing. I am ravenously hungry virtually 100 percent of the time, so I spend a great deal of my workday walking methodically around the office, like Arnold Schwarzenegger in "The Terminator," searching for a leftover pizza crust or some other pathetic morsel of food. The result is that whenever there are any leftovers floating around the office, they generally find their way in my direction.

Which is great, except that it always seems to happen when I am about to leave for a serious workout. It never happens when I've run 10 miles that morning and am so monstrously hungry that I'm starting to salt my Post-It Notes. And it always poses an extremely difficult test of my moral character. Do I tearfully pass on the ice cream cake, knowing full well that later on when I am desperate for nourishment there will be nothing around except ketchup packets, or do I wolf the thing down knowing that I will be cursing myself an hour later as I'm burping my way around the track?

What I've learned over the years is that the key to maintaining control over your workout schedule is to treat your relationship with your workout much the same way you would treat any other key relationship in your life. You simply can't let on how important it is to you, or it will destroy you. You have to play it casual. Your attitude has to be something along the lines of, "Gee, it would be nice if I could get a couple miles in sometime this afternoon, but if not, no big deal, there's always another day." You've got to approach it this way even when you're really sitting at your desk thinking, "If I don't get out there today and run 10 hard miles at a 6:30 pace, I am going to pull my eyebrows out with this staple remover." Because if you let on how much it means to you, guaranteed that when you go unpack your gym bag, you'll find two left shoes.

Meanwhile, I am sorry to report that I am experiencing some difficulties in my relationship with my current workout. I was supposed to go for a nice long run later this evening. But I just can't tonight. I have a headache.

From Oxygen Debt to Training Bankruptcy

It all began innocently enough. It was a Wednesday, and my training schedule called for a long afternoon run. But I was busy at work, the weather was lousy, one of my socks had a hole in it — all the usual lame-excuse suspects — and so, in a moment of weakness, I gave in to temptation: I took out a workout loan.

I decided it was OK to blow off the run if I promised myself I would repay the loan in full the next day by running during my lunch hour and still doing my regular Thursday night swim workout. Little did I know I was mortgaging my training future. In the first place, this required some highly questionable accounting practices in my training log. I'm not proud of it, but I must confess that I pre-entered the next day's run. I recognize this is a clear violation of generally accepted Training Log Practices, which require that workouts actually be completed prior to log entry.

In my own defense, I figured that if I wrote the run down in my log, I would have no choice about actually doing it the next day. After all, it's already in the log. And once I actually did the workout, there would be no harm done. This kind of reasoning has launched many a career in white-collar crime. If I'm ever the target of a workout audit, I'll probably be convicted on several counts of mile fraud.

My cooking of the books boiled over the very next day, Thursday, when I got sent out of town on business, forcing me to miss both the repayment of my run loan and my regular swim workout. All of a sudden, I was two workouts in the red, and starting to panic. As a result of my frantic efforts to pay off the mounting debt by squeezing in extra workouts, I didn't have enough time left over to meet my regular training obligations as they came due. I was in a downward spiral toward total workout insolvency.

This crisis could have been averted if there were an open market in which triathletes could trade workouts like commodities. If you were short a swim one week, but had an extra couple of running miles, you could hire a workout broker to find someone who needed to pick up a quick run and was willing to make you a deal on a decent pool workout.

There are a lot of possibilities here. Triathletes who train like maniacs and are always ahead of their weekly goals could sell their extra mileage for some much-needed cash. You could even try your luck by speculating on workout futures. If you sensed a nasty week of weather approaching, you could stockpile bike workouts, then sit back, wait for prices to rise and make a killing.

But with the market not being an option, I finally had to admit that I was in over my head, and that there was only one way out: declare total training bankruptcy. I had to suffer the humiliation of a total training reorganization, in which some of my unpaid workouts were written off entirely, while others were sold off at discounted rates — a 100-yard sprint for every running mile skipped; 25 yards of freestyle for every missed 100 IM.

Now, my overall workout portfolio has been sharply cut back, I have trouble getting new training partners, and I feel a deep sense of personal shame. All because of that innocent little workout loan I thought I'd have no trouble paying off. I am hoping my sad example will be a warning for some of you, and that maybe some good will come of it. Take it from me: Don't give in to temptation, or you may find yourself in a workout hole so deep you'll never be able to swim, bike or run your way out of it. And invest wisely in your workout future. If you find yourself with a couple extra hours on a Sunday afternoon, get in a quick 40-mile ride, even if it's not on your schedule. You'll be putting something away for, literally, a rainy day.

Swim, Bike, Run... Zzzzzzzzz

It has always amused me — and I'm sure it has sent my bosses over the years into absolute hysterics — that people think because I do an occasional triathlon I must be a highly motivated, super energetic, Type-A freak. The fact is that when I'm not out there racing or training, I rank, in terms of general alertness and get-up-and-go, somewhere just below your average course monitor in the fourth hour of an Olympic-distance triathlon.

How lazy am I? Consider this: I had one of those runs the other day during which a toenail — and I'm not one to name toes — committed a vicious, unprovoked assault on a neighboring toe. Even though all toes could have stood a trimming, I could only muster the energy to cut that one nail — leaving discipline of the other toes for a later time when they, too, turned violent. In that sense it was very much like our criminal justice system.

But the point is not to illustrate my shortcomings in personal hygiene — that's an issue for another chapter. The point is that triathletes are pretty good when it comes to physical energy, but when it comes to mental effort, sometimes we struggle. Some days, sitting at my desk in the office, I need to summon every ounce of strength just to press the keys on my keyboard far enough to convince the computer that I'm serious. It can get so bad that I have to let my body go limp, prop my chin on a pencil to keep my head from rolling over, and channel all remaining energy into my fingertips.

But if someone were to come into my office for a quick mid-morning run, I'd be bounding out the door like a cartoon character. And I see this same behavior in many of my triathlon friends. I think what's happened is that all the training has caused a chemical mutation whereby our brains can function only when our heart rates are above 155. We've become life-sized wind-up toys, like those little kids' robots that light up and wave their arms and generally go berserk when you roll them along the floor, but go dead the second you stop. The result is that our lives become a repeating pattern of short bursts of insanely vigorous activity, followed by extended periods of almost complete dormancy. *That* bodes well for our futures.

It's comforting to think that it's the constant training that deprives our brains of the oxygen necessary to focus on other aspects of our lives — jobs, relationships, finances, minor details like that — and that if we just ditched the training, we'd be as diligent as the next guy. But sometimes I worry it might be the other way around. I think we train like lunatics in a desperate attempt to compensate for the laziness we exhibit in the rest of our lives. The basic, twisted reasoning goes something like this: OK, I got nothing done at work today, didn't finish that damn report and I'm much too lazy to pay the bills, balance my checkbook or do the laundry. But I did crank out a hard, 10-mile run — in the rain — SO I MUST BE A GOOD PERSON! Admit it: It takes a lot less mental energy to jump in the pool for a 3000-yard workout than to finish those cover letters or that stupid tax return.

I should probably write some more about this very important issue, but it's been a couple of hours since my last workout, and the mind's starting to wander. I think it's time for a bike ride.

Chapter 4

Swim

Pond Scum

Sometimes you've really got to wonder about the humans. A while back, for example, I was out for a bike ride with some friends in rural Massachusetts, when we stumbled on an awesome little pond. There was a beach at one end with some people scattered around and a couple lifeguards up on stands, so we wandered over, parked our bikes, grabbed some goggles out of our packs and waded in for a little swim.

A very small area of the pond had been roped off with a line of buoys. But the buoys didn't extend more than about 15 yards from the shore, and I figured they were there just to keep the little kids under wraps, so we stepped over the rope and started to swim out into the open water.

Well, if you've had much experience dealing with the humans, I bet you can predict what happened next. As soon as we got past the rope line, what seemed like the entire Massachusetts law enforcement community came down on us like we were international terrorists. Park rangers came chasing after us in a motor boat. A police helicopter with a searchlight hovered overhead. A guy on shore in a suit and tie got out a bullhorn to try to talk us back in.

OK, maybe I exaggerate. But if we had set up a little stand on the beach selling crack to the schoolchildren, I doubt we would have met with such a swift and stern response. I couldn't believe they were serious. I kid you not, at its deepest point there was no more than a foot-and-a-half of water within the roped-off area. You couldn't actually swim within the buoys without having your bathing suit fill up with silt from scraping the bottom of the pond. The lifeguards were wearing polo shirts and khakis, with the cuffs rolled up below their knees in case they actually had to perform a daring rescue.

It seems the job of lifeguard has changed considerably from when we were kids. Instead of preventing people from getting hurt while swimming, now the job seems to be to prevent them from swimming at all. As explained to me afterward by one of the rangers (he was not a Power Ranger, it turns out, just a regular old ranger, and he did not seem at all amused by the question), it is *extremely* illegal to swim outside the roped off area in Massachusetts ponds. I was very lucky to get off with just a warning, he said, because ordinarily the offense carries a six-year prison sentence, plus a public spanking.

I simply cannot imagine who in his or her right mind would take a perfect little pond, and go and ruin it like this. It's like serving a beautiful pizza in an Italian restaurant, and then marking off a small segment of crust and announcing that the rest of the pie is off-limits to eating. If they had told me that I was swimming at my own risk outside the ropes, that they weren't going to get their khakis wet trying to save me if I got into trouble, that's cool, I could live with that (so to speak). But to actually make swimming in the pond *illegal?*

You have to wonder about the deliberative process behind a piece of legislation like this. I imagine it probably went something like this down at the State House in Boston:

> *First lawmaker:* We have a problem with the ponds. People are swimming in them!
>
> *Second lawmaker:* My god! They must be stopped!
>
> *Third lawmaker:* I'll have another Guinness!
>
> *First lawmaker:* Then it's unanimous! Moving on, we have reports that people are actually hiking on the trails!
>
> *Second lawmaker:* The heathens!
>
> *Third lawmaker:* Burp.

The problem, of course, is that your average politician is generally not an avid participant in recreational sports, at least those not involving inappropriate sexual contact with an intern, while the typical athlete usually has little time or patience for politics, and so we're extremely underrepresented in the political process, which is why we end up getting barred from swimming in our own ponds.

The solution is to get more involved in educating our elected officials. And so, as a public service, I've prepared the following handy little chart, which I hope will at least be a step in the right direction:

Crime	Not a Crime
Murder	Swimming
Robbery	Biking
Embezzlement	Running

Perhaps we can post this in state houses across the country. And while we're at it, we've got to get the government to do something about those rollerbladers. Those people are a menace. They should be outlawed.

The Swim Coach

OK, I'm sure hockey coaches are very much into hockey, football coaches live and breathe football, and basketball coaches dream about the perfect man-to-man full-court trap. But seriously, I don't know why, but somehow swim coaches are just . . . different. In my experience, most of them have done one flip-turn too many, if you know what I mean.

For many years, I swam with a group that met every Sunday night at a pool in rural Connecticut. Our swim coach was an extremely earnest, endearing, 50ish guy with long, whitish, chlorine-damaged hair whose entire mission in life, God bless him, was to get us to rotate our hips to lengthen our freestyle stroke.

Every Sunday we would have a "classroom session" before our swim workout. My favorite part of class was when Coach decided that he had seized on an aspect of swim technique so critical that it required an immediate visual demonstration. This was when Coach, without a moment's hesitation, would dive belly-down on the cold linoleum classroom floor to demonstrate the proper elbow bend during the recovery phase of the stroke, while the rest of us gathered round and watched apprehensively, like a crowd watching a stranger go into cardiac arrest at the Mall.

Because Coach believed that visualization is critical to mastering proper swim technique, he liked to show us an instructional swimming video during each Sunday night session before we jumped in the pool. Sounds sensible, right? Again, you have underestimated the long-term effects of chlorine saturation. The problem was that Coach had only one video.

I am not making this up. Each Sunday for the better part of a decade, Coach would announce with great fanfare that he had a videotape that will really help us understand the techniques he'd been trying to instill. And each Sunday we'd all exchange furtive glances and think to ourselves, OK, this has *got* to be a new one, right? Anything else would be insane. And each Sunday it would be the exact same thing. You know how some people have seen Sylvester Stallone in *Rocky* like 57 times? Well, I have seen Rowdy Gaines in *Basic Technique from the Fast Lane* at least 127 times.

And it's not like there's a shortage of swimming videos. These days you can find three-volume instructional DVDs devoted entirely to proper thumb positioning during the entry phase of the stroke. It seems like every former college swimmer has tried to delay the inevitability of getting a Real Job by launching a series of "How To Improve Your Swim Stroke" videotapes. I enjoy watching these videos not so much for their instructional value as for their amusement value. They all have a certain bad-porn-video production quality to them —poor lighting, shaky camera work, nondescript hotel room setting, excessive nudity — and they all feature a very embarrassed-looking young person stand-ing around in a Speedo while the swimming "expert" manipulates his or her limbs in cruel and humiliating ways to demonstrate proper form. I always imagine that this swimmer has agreed to the assignment for a little extra credit in her phys ed class, and will live to regret it, like a struggling actress who poses nude in search of her big break.

Anyway, after our classroom session it was into the pool for our actual workout, and I've got to hand it to Coach, he was right in there with us. To pick up flaws in our stroke, Coach would float eerily at the bottom of the pool, like the floating bodies in the movie *Coma*, and study our technique as we swam over him. When he spotted something he didn't like, he would lunge at us, shark-attack like, seize our elbow or foot or whatever the offend-ing body part happened to be, and physically correct the defect right there on the spot.

I am willing to admit that swimming is a highly technical sport, but sometimes you really have to wonder whether mastering all of these tiny technical details is worth the effort. I have been swim-ming for a while now, I have tried S-pulls and reverse-S pulls, I have tried two-beat kicks and four-beat kicks and ska-beat kicks, and I think maybe over the years I have gotten my 100 time down from 1:17 to about 1:16.7. Sometimes I think every one of us has a built-in swimming coefficient, which pretty much determines how fast we're going to swim, technique or no technique, which explains why I can be in the pool with my high elbows and relaxed recovery and still get passed by guys swimming like Curly from the Three Stooges.

Incidentally, I hear that Curly is coming out with a new swim-ming video. Someone please send it to my swim coach.

Swimming Circles Around the Issues

Politicians are always yammering about things like health care reform and balancing the federal budget, but if you ask me, no issue cries out more for national attention than swimming pool etiquette.

One issue that needs to be addressed right at the outset is the pre-swim shower. Maybe I'm off the deep end here, but I just don't see the need to stand under a shower before jumping into a swimming pool, and frankly I'm always a little bit offended by those signs demanding showers before entering the pool area. Those signs must be left over from days when people got a whole lot dirtier than they do now. If I had just come from a day in the mines, and I was caked head to toe in soot, then I could see how a shower would be reasonable. But given that I'm an attorney, and I only get covered in filth in a metaphorical sense, taking a shower before a swim seems redundant. I imagine these signs are made by the same company that makes the placards in restaurant bathrooms reminding employees to wash their hands after use (after use of what, I always wonder). Hopefully, the restaurant signs have a far greater level of compliance than the swimming pool signs. Why doesn't this company quit pestering swimmers, who are generally a fairly clean group to begin with, and start making signs requiring showers in places where they'll be more useful? Like before boarding an airplane.

Another divisive swimming-pool-related issue is the matter of splitting versus circling. Studies have proven that two swimmers alone in a lane will almost always conspire to split it, regardless of the circumstances. Swimmers are such dreamers. Even if a half dozen swimmers are standing pool-side, spitting in their goggles and toeing the water, the swimmers in the pool will cling desperately to the romantic vision of a split lane. All this does, of course, is set the stage for trouble when the inevitable third swimmer enters the picture.

It seems to me that both the new entrants and the incumbent swimmers have responsibilities here. It seems obvious that the new entrant cannot simply jump in and begin doing circles without alerting the pre-existing swimmers. This is a bit like taking the wrong on-ramp onto a highway on the assumption that all the other cars will automatically switch over to driving on the left. Yet we all know from experience that this happens with alarming frequency in a pool.

I am not sure what the new entrants are thinking. Perhaps their theory is that the swimmers already in the pool will pick up on subtle changes in the Doppler effect and modify their patterns accordingly. Maybe someone ought to test their blood-chlorine levels. But the new entrants do not shoulder sole responsibility for the split-circle transition. The incumbent swimmers have an obligation as well. It is an all-too-familiar tactic among some veteran swimmers to feign ignorance of a new arrival, disregarding all efforts to alert them to the population change, in the desperate hope that maybe the newcomer will give up and pick another lane that's a little easier to break into. Swimmers will do anything to avoid even the slightest disruption to their workout, because, as we all know, if you're trying to do a set of 100s on 1:30, and some lane disturbance forces you to start one on 1:32, the whole set is void and you have to start over. I have seen swimmers so determined to appear unaware of a new lane arrival that it would have taken a harpoon to stop them from flip-turning right on through.

Once a new swimmer has been assimilated into the lane and a circling regime has been established, that simply presents another, and perhaps even graver, problem: Inevitably, the new swimmer is going to be doing 1500 yards of sidestroke. It would be nice if swimmers in the same lane were close to the same pace, but we simply are not organized enough as a species to make this happen. Perhaps, in the future, every swimmer should be required to swim a qualifying lap, like at the Indy 500, so they can be placed in the appropriate lane. But until then, there will always be swimmers who believe it is their divine right to float on their backs in the interval training lane, so there is really no getting around the issue of passing.

As triathletes, we're all accustomed to a fair amount of physical contact in the water — there's more body contact at the start of a triathlon than in your average NBA playoff game — but your generic pool swimmer is often taken aback by this. So, regrettably, swimming directly over the top of slower swimmers is probably out of line. Which leaves you two options: the toe tap, or passing down the center. Both have their pros and cons. The toe tap, of course, requires the cooperation of the slower swimmer, and I'm sure I am not the only one to hypothesize that the obliviousness of a swimmer often seems to be inversely proportional to his or her speed. (A dead swimmer, for example, has maximum obliviousness and minimum speed, so the theory seems to test out at the extremes.) This would make the down-the-middle option the more desirable of the two, except for the fact that it requires the passing swimmer to make some very complex calculations, including (a) the distance between him/herself and the wall; (b) the relative speeds of him/herself and the slow swimmer, and (c) the pros and cons of calling it a day and going for a beer. Let me just say, in passing, that the beer solution is almost always my personal preference.

Surf Battles

So I'm in the middle of a swim workout at my club the other night, when all of a sudden, I'm getting tangled in the lane line like a dolphin caught in a tuna fishing net. This can be an extremely startling and disorienting feeling, for both dolphins and humans. At first I thought I'd lost concentration and veered off course a bit, so I made a slight correction, but then there's the rope line still right in my face. My next thought was that I'm having some kind of neurological incident that is causing me to lose all sense of direction and that I'm almost certainly going to drown, which is going to put a serious crimp in my training.

But, of course, it turned out to be just the water aerobics people again. Several times a week, one-half of my club's lap pool is reserved for a relatively new form of physical exercise known as "water aerobics." For the convenience of the other health club members, these sessions are always kept on a regular schedule, which is described in the health club calendar as "whenever there happens to be enough people hanging around with nothing better to do than water aerobics."

Of course, the water aerobics people cannot be bothered with actually speaking to the lap swimmers. (And I have to admit that, in my case, this is probably a wise decision, as you may be able to guess from the tone of this chapter.) Instead, they opt to simply untie the lane lines and haul them out of the pool, raking them across the heads and bodies of the swimmers in the process, on the theory that sooner or later the swimmers will either drown or get out of the way. It's usually a pretty effective technique, causing the swimmers to migrate simultaneously to the other half of the pool, cursing like sailors all the way, like some very poorly choreographed and profane synchronized swimming routine, and then try to integrate with the other swimmers who had been happily occupying the "aerobics-free" half of the pool.

In my opinion, this is a significant amount of chaos to be inflicted by an activity that, as far as I can tell, offers no shred of aerobic or any other recognizable physiological benefit. Now I recognize that this is exactly the kind of intolerant and condescending attitude that gives triathletes a bad name, and I agree that we should be supportive of everyone's effort to improve their fitness levels, regardless of how ludicrous and annoying it may be. But seriously, water aerobics? Perhaps some water aerobics classes offer a vigorous cardiovascular workout, but at my club, the class consists of absolutely nothing more than bobbing in the pool like water lilies in a pond, with an occasional tidal migration from one end of the pool to the other. There is no doubt in my mind that Monet would get more exercise *painting* the water aerobics class than the participants are getting by actually engaging in it. Maybe as a complement to the water aerobics program, and to alleviate overcrowding in the pool, the health club should introduce a new program called "air swimming," in which the participants congregate in the aerobics studio and, under the guidance of an experienced air swimming instructor, simulate various swim strokes for an hour.

What really gets my heart rate up is when the water aerobicists decide to bring their children to the pool with them, on the theory that they can get their "workout" in and give their kids a chance to frolic in the pool at the very same time. The result, of course, is that not only are all the actual swimmers crammed into half as many lanes, but they also spend much of their time swimming into floating pails, shovels, water wings and even the occasional small child who plunges into the water directly in a swimmer's path. It always amazes me how oblivious the water aerobicists are to the complete havoc their children are causing, and the visible rage welling up inside the swimmers. The few times I've stopped my workout to shoot a clearly hostile stare in their direction, they always have a cluelessly blissful smile on their bloated bobbing faces that says, "Isn't it wonderful to see the children having such fun?"

I have a solution to propose, and I think it's a reasonable one. All I ask is that these people and their children never be permitted to set foot in a swimming facility for the remainder of their lives. If that is viewed by the mainstream population as too extreme, then I also have a backup plan, and suffice it to say it involves a tuna fishing net.

Hotel Hell

How many times has this happened to you: You're traveling on business and desperate for a workout. You check into your $249-a-night hotel, and you're thrilled to learn from the desk clerk that the hotel does in fact have a fitness center. So you dump your bags in your room and change into your workout clothes . . . only to discover that the fitness center used to be Room 837 until they dragged in two rusty stationary bikes and a Universal set from 1985. Basically, the hotel has spent more money on the drapes in your room than on the entire fitness center.

I always wonder how they picked Room 837. I figure some very unfortunate event must have taken place in that room that left it particularly malodorous, and they couldn't figure out what to do with it until some hotel exec said, "Hey, let's have a fitness center!" Unfortunately, the room wasn't quite big enough, making it physically impossible to do most of the exercises on the Universal without sledgehammering down one of the walls, which would probably result in an entry on your hotel bill even larger than making a long-distance phone call. And if you're planning on riding the stationary bike, I hope you brought your own toe clips. Clearly someone has traveled the world stealing toe clips out of hotel gyms, and now has the world's largest toe-clip collection in his or her basement. Personally, I don't travel anywhere without my own personal toe-clip set. And don't ask me where I got them.

Then there is the whole matter of the hotel pool. Hotel operators have discovered that if people actually swim in their pools, this increases the risk that someone might drown, and so their pools have been skillfully engineered to make them virtually impossible to swim in. You can forget about lane lines, and I wonder how much time was spent in the lab to develop a color of paint that makes the pool walls completely invisible when viewed from under water. Not only aren't hotel pools rectangular, they aren't even kidney shaped, which is usually the bodily organ of choice when it comes to pool shapes. I guess the pool engineers decided that swimmers have figured out the kidney, so most hotel pools are now shaped like far more exotic and complex organs such as the esophagus. (Please don't waste your time emailing me that the esophagus isn't technically an organ. Tell it to the swimming pool manufacturers.)

Absolutely true story: I stayed at a hotel in Florida a while back and was stunned to look out my hotel room window and see a gorgeous, rectangular, 25-yard outdoor pool, complete with lane lines. The only thing standing in the way of an awesome workout was a line of buoys running straight across the middle of the pool, perpendicular to the lanes. I figured I could easily unhook the buoys and get in a good 10- or 15-minute swim before hotel security swooped down on me like paratroopers. When I got down to the pool, however, I discovered — I am not making this up — that the buoy line was permanently welded to the pool walls. I would have needed a blowtorch to get it off. It was as if, at the very last minute, the pool engineers looked at each other and said, "Wait a minute! Do you think someone might actually try to *swim* in this pool??"

Even if you can get past all these structural difficulties, you then have to deal with the fact that, by statute, hotel pools are required to be occupied round-the-clock by families from Iowa or, in some jurisdictions, from Hell. These families have an average of 47 children and appear to have never seen a swimming pool before in their lives, and as a result are so excited that they feel obliged to conduct all of their daily activities in the water, including getting dressed in the morning, barbecuing dinner, and other activities that I would prefer not to even think about. Why these people aren't at Disney World, instead of a Hyatt in New Jersey, is a complete mystery to me.

If you take all of these factors — the esophagus-shaped pool, no lane lines, the family from Hell, etc. — and insert a triathlete in Speedo and goggles attempting to do a workout, you end up with a scene right out of one of those Which-Object-Does-Not-Belong-In-This-Picture games from an old *Highlights* magazine. The only real question at this point is which object you're going to swim into first: a small Midwestern child, a floating barbecue grill, or, if you're lucky enough to make it all the way across, the pool wall.

Chapter 5

Bike

Bike Technology Made Simple

Bicycle technology has gotten so complex lately that I thought I would take a moment to pass along the benefits of my knowledge and expertise on the subject.

There are basically three broad species of bicycle in existence today: "road bikes," which are built to be light and aerodynamic for long rides on flat surfaces; "mountain bikes," which are built to be tough and durable for riding up mountains and over rocks and tree stumps; and "hybrid bikes," which are built to do neither. Naturally, hybrids have been far and away the most popular species of bikes among consumers over the past few decades.

The bicycle itself can be broken down into the "frame," which is self-explanatory, and the "components." Bicycle components are very intricate and complex and intimidating and nobody really understands how they work, so you don't need to worry too much about them. All you need to know is that all of them are made by either "Campagnolo" or "Shimano." Campagnolo prefers to go by its nickname, "Campy," but when you are angry with a Campy component you should of course address it by its full name, as in, "All right, Campagnolo, you had better shift into third gear *right now.*"

Which brings us to perhaps the most popular but least understood and certainly the most frequently misspelled component, the "derailleur," which comes from the French word "de-," meaning "rarely," and "railleur," meaning "works." The derailleur's job is pretty simple: shift the chain from one gear to another. Unfortunately, some derailleurs approach their jobs like entry-level workers at large corporations: They have a very simple job to do, a job that is quite frankly well beneath their ability level, which creates a serious motivational problem and causes them to perform their assigned task in an extremely careless and slovenly manner, such as, for example, ignoring specific instructions from the rider to shift to a particular gear, and then later switching without notice to a random gear based on nothing more than their own whim and caprice.

Campagnolo and Shimano make about 167,000 different "groups" of components, with very helpful explanatory names like "Athena," "Chorus," "Deore," "Ultegra" and my own personal favorite, "Dura-Ace," giving cyclists a lot of options to decide how much they want to spend. This has always seemed a bit strange. Since the derailleur exists to perform one very simple task — to shift gears — it seems to me that the only conceivable difference between all these derailleur groups is that some actually *can* shift your gears. You shouldn't really have to pay extra for that.

Buying a new bike these days can be a bit overwhelming because it seems like there are dozens of different bike manufacturers to choose from. But it turns out it isn't all that complicated, because all these manufacturers are actually owned by a single company called Trek, which also owns General Motors and has a permanent seat on the United Nations Security Council. Rumor has it that Trek and Shimano are planning to merge and come out with a new brand of bike called "Shmek," which by total coincidence turns out to be the Yiddish word for "extremely expensive bicycle."

Sizing is very important when buying a new bike, because if your bike doesn't fit you properly, you will be uncomfortable and, worse, you will look goofy riding it. In order to get the proper fit, it is critical to get professionally "sized" on a bike, which requires you to attempt to balance yourself in an undignified manner on an immobile bicycle in the middle of a crowded bike shop while the salespeople and all the other shoppers stand around and laugh at you. The bicycle manufacturers have made the sizing process easier for you by randomly alternating between centimeters and inches when measuring the key dimensions on the bicycle, and sometimes both at the same time, so that you have to ask for inner tubes in sizes like 700cm x 1 ½ inches, even though you have no idea what any of those numbers mean. My strategy is to grab a couple of tube boxes off the shelf and get out of the bike store as quickly as possible, before a sales clerk asks me a highly technical question I have no idea how to answer, like what size my wheels are.

Which, by the way, is something that happens frequently, because bike people are always sniffing around each other's bikes like dogs in a park on Sunday morning, asking all kinds of questions about mechanical aspects of my bike that I really couldn't care less about, like what kind of "fork" I have. When this happens I usually resort to an old trick I learned practicing law, which is to make stuff up, so I will mutter something about how I'm trying out the new synthetic onyx fork that I'm sure they've heard about, and then ride off as quickly as possible.

Another important variable is the composition of the frame. There are several different substances out there all vying to be *your* frame substance. The traditional ones are steel and aluminum, and the exotic newer substances are "carbon fiber," which can also be found in many brands of breakfast cereal, and titanium, which I used to think was a completely fictional substance but is actually a high-tech material used only in bicycle frames and nuclear reactors. Each of these substances is said to have its own unique "feel," and I'm sure this would be true if you were, for example, chewing on it; but when it comes to bikes, frankly I doubt anyone can really tell the difference.

To sum up, if you're looking to buy a new bike, I recommend that you do what the experts do, which is to read up on all the latest technology, test ride as many different types of bikes as possible, and then, in the end, buy the one that you think looks the coolest.

Car Wars

It's very hard to remain optimistic about human nature when you commute to work by bike. I'd be willing to bet that whoever started the old philosophical debate about whether humans are inherently good or inherently evil never tried to ride a bike down a city street at rush hour. It would take about a block and a half to convince even the most soft-hearted philosopher that not only are humans inherently evil, they're inherently homicidal.

It's funny how you can always tell the real psychos a mile away. I don't know whether it's the Darth Vader-like tint to their windshields, or the evil hum coming from their engines, or what, but you can sense them, like bad guys in a Western movie. Does this sound familiar: You're riding down the right-hand side of the right lane of a fairly busy road, minding your own business. One by one, the cars coming up in the right lane behind you are faced with the decision of how to get by, and generally they seem to handle it OK. True, occasionally you get one that hovers nervously behind you, too timid to pass, probably thinking they're being extraordinarily courteous to you when in fact they're driving you NUTS and making you wish they'd just mow you down already to end the tension. But apart from that, by and large most drivers seem to handle this situation without too much angst.

Until, that is, you hear the evil hum, and you know you've got one of THEM behind you. Invariably they'll VROOM up next to you, pause there menacingly just to let you know that they're not going to kill you this time but they could have if they'd wanted to, and probably will if you have the audacity to do this again, and then they'll VROOM off dramatically into the distance, presumably to demonstrate the vast technological superiority of their combustion engine to your pathetic chainring . . . until, of course, you pass them 200 yards later at the next red light. And tell the truth, is there a cyclist among us who can resist the smug little wave?

Or how about this: You're riding the "discouraged" way down a one-way street, but you're keeping a nice tight line on the right-hand side, and it's a wide one-way street, a one-way street that really would have served just fine as a two-wayer if some civil engineer hadn't read too many Games magazines, when up ahead you see that Darth Vader windshield coming at you. Right away you can tell you're dealing with someone who's had a bad day, if not life. Even though there's plenty of room to pass on by, Darth will invariably exercise his God-given vehicular right to occupy the extreme left-most region of the roadway, to demonstrate the mayhem that you're causing by going the wrong way on what, he will loudly educate you as he passes angrily by, is a ONE-WAY STREET! And then he'll lop off your front wheel with his light saber.

Misanthropy, however, is not the only side-effect of commuting by bike. My favorite side-effect occurs when I make the unfortunate error of getting behind the wheel of an actual car. When you're used to the relative freedom of the bicycle, traffic laws become more like . . . what's the right word . . . *guidelines*. A red light doesn't mean "stop" as much as "stop if some object will actually strike you if you attempt to cross at this instant, otherwise go for it." A "one-way" sign means "one way, unless this happens to be the most direct way to get where you're going, in which case you'd have to be a total moron to go any other way."

From what I understand, however, when you're driving an actual car, these signs are meant to be taken literally, even if they produce absolutely absurd results, like forcing you to come to a complete stop and just SIT THERE at a red light even though NO ONE'S COMING!! I am not very good at this, and there have been many occasions when I've been at a red light and caught myself an instant before reflexively darting through a break in the traffic.

Parking creates similar problems. When you're on your bike, the only obstacle to parking is the geometric complexity of getting that U-lock around the parking meter and your wheel and your frame, which often seems as impossible as those irritating little untangling brain-teaser games people always have on their coffee tables. And it's even tougher when your bike is being uncooperative. Tell me if I'm wrong about this, but it seems like sometimes your handlebars will be barely grazing a tree branch and the bike will stand at attention like a soldier at roll call, and other times you can prop it firmly against a wall, with everything you know about physics and gravity telling you it ought to stay right there, and it'll keep squirming to the ground like a whiny three-year-old. Bikes are so moody that way.

But the point is that, minor inconveniences aside, when you're on your bike you don't have to give parking a second thought; you just ride on up to the front of where you're going and you're done. Which is why I'm terrified that one day I'll be leaving a restaurant, and there will be a commotion out front, and I'll discover that I've absent-mindedly driven up on the curb and Kryptonited my car to a lamppost. I wonder what the fine is for that.

Re-Cycling Catalogues

You can find them in every nook and cranny of my house. On the bathroom floor, in a big pile in the corner of my study, strewn all over the coffee table in my living room. No, I'm not talking about old running shoes, although that's a very good guess. I'm talking about magazines. And not even old *Sports Illustrateds* or *National Geographics*, like a normal person. I'm talking about cycling catalogues.

It seems like I get a new catalogue at least once a day, the late-summer issue, the really-late-summer issue, the ok-we'll-pay-you-to-order-some-of-this-leftover-crap issue. And even though these catalogues are basically all interchangeable going back thousands of years, for some reason I can never bring myself to throw the old ones away. I suppose you never know when you might want to research the sale price of marble handlebar tape back in August 1998. The result is that they're strewn in piles all over my apartment, like some bizarre neon-colored high-gloss mineral deposit. This can be a major health hazard, because the cycling catalogue is one of the slipperiest objects known to man. Hit one of those babies on the floor in your bare feet and it's all over. Forget Pam at your next race, just slip a couple old catalogues up the leg of your wetsuit and it'll slide right off.

But I have to admit that the cycling catalogue can be a uniquely entertaining piece of American literature. First of all, have you ever studied the facial expressions on the models in the typical bike catalogue? I'm guessing that this has to be the single lowest rung on the fashion modeling ladder. They all look more or less embarrassed to be there. And who can blame them? It is extremely difficult to look anything other than absolutely ridiculous posing in a pair of bib shorts. I can just imagine an agent having to break the news to her client:

> *Agent:* Hey, guess what, you got your first model-ing job!
>
> *Model:* Wow, that's great!! What is it, Vogue? Cosmo?
>
> *Agent:* Not exactly. . .

Model: OK then, what??

Agent: Um . . . well, the good news is, they're going
to throw in a free water bottle cage!

I can't imagine it's all that exciting being a photographer for
a cycling catalogue either. It's not exactly like landing the *Sports
Illustrated* swimsuit gig. I mean, how much can you do with a pair
of thermal fleece gloves . . . maybe airbrush out the lint stuck in
the velcro strap? Just once, I would like to open my mailbox and
see the new Victoria's Secret cycling catalogue. Personally, I think
the Miracle Tri-Suit would be a top seller.

My favorite part of the cycling catalogue is toward the back,
where you get into the real hard-core gear, the hubs and forks
and headset spacers and bar ends and whirlygigs and gizmos of
every shape and description. I love the helpful charts they put in
there to explain the subtle variations between the models. I'm
convinced they make most of the categories up. A typical chart
looks like this:

Item	Vertical Weight	Viscosity	SDP	Itch Gradient
A. HP7-AX	13.4g	427 pdi	under	6 LEQs
B. HP7-AY	13.6g	6,987 pdi	over	10 LEQs
C. 12LCX	12.3g	548 pdi	over/under	7.5 LEQs

And that's just for a pair of socks. They get a little carried away
with the trademarks in the catalogues as well. I understand that it
can be difficult to distinguish one taillight from another, but really,
Super Nebula Cosmic Whitelight XRay 5000 XL2001? Isn't that
maybe just a little over the top?

The Real Information Superhighway

All anyone ever talks about these days is the Internet, and frankly, I'm getting sick of it. It's not that I don't appreciate the fact that modern technology now makes it possible that, by noon on Sunday, the entire known universe can find out how slowly I raced that morning. It's just that in all this hype over the 'Net, I think we've overlooked another communications breakthrough that might be just as important, although admittedly much more low tech.

The magnitude of this alternative social network was revealed to me last weekend, when I went for a bike ride with a friend who was training for one of those cycling fund raisers that are popping up all over the place. There are so many of these things nowadays that you can pretty much sit on a bike and fund-raise 24 hours a day, 365 days a year, coast-to-coast, without ever paying for your own Gatorade or energy bars. . . provided, of course, that you have enough friends to constantly hit up for $10 apiece.

Anyway, the organizers of this particular event decided to stage helpful little training rides to get participants ready for the Big Day. They held these training events on the actual course, and because the course maps hadn't been printed yet, they marked the course with cute little yellow arrows to guide riders in the right direction. On this particular day, we were the only riders who elected to take advantage of this training opportunity. This is because most normal people understood that it would be just as effective to go out and do *any* 50 mile ride; we didn't need to drive an hour to ride the actual 50-mile course. But my friend, an extremely enthusiastic beginning cyclist doing her first organized event, decided that it was imperative to go out and ride the exact, authentic 50 miles that the organizers had staked out, or she wouldn't be properly prepared.

OK, fine. Of course, because there was no map and no other riders on the course, we spent the next several hours riding around, staring intently and neurotically at the pavement, terrified that we would miss an arrow and bike off the edge of a cliff or something. This made for a very stressful ride. Turns out that it's pretty easy to miss a six-inch yellow chalk arrow at 25 mph, and so I was constantly doubling back for missed turns, like a Pac-Man character from that old video game.

But during this ordeal, I began to notice the huge volume of communication taking place on the pavement beneath me. In addition to our little arrows, there were blue arrows, red arrows, squiggly arrows, arrows with initials, arrows with little smiley faces on them, all remnants of some past (or for all I knew, future) event.

And it wasn't just the cyclists who were using the roads as their own private message board. The road runners had their courses marked out, too; construction crews had messages and measurements stenciled all over the roads to commemorate the last time they'd gnarled traffic to lay a piece of pipe; and the local high school kids left messages of various degrees of literacy and obscenity to memorialize practically every event in their daily lives. The net result was an incredibly complex maze of messages, the modern equivalent of the ancient cave drawings you'd see in *National Geographic*.

It occurred to me that we ought to embrace this new medium with the same capitalist gusto with which the rest of the world is embracing the Internet. The marketing geniuses at Performance and Nashbar and Pearl Izumi ought to be out there painting ads on the blacktop like there's no tomorrow. Newspaper publishers, desperate to reach new audiences, should spray-paint the morning's headlines at key intersections for diehard cyclists who are on the road at 6 a.m. and don't have time to read the morning paper. If this catches on, maybe they'll replace the yellow lines with those electronic message screens, like on elevators in big office buildings, so cyclists can have news, weather and sports scrolling under their wheels 24 hours a day. That way, we won't miss as much by doing those year-round fund-raisers.

Well, that's it for now, I've got to run. I've got a blind date with a girl who answered the personal ad I spray-painted at the 25-mile mark out on Old Country Road.

Who needs Facebook?

Nevermore, Dude

Once upon a midday dreary, while I pedaled, weak and weary,
Over many a quaint and curious mile of forgotten ore —
While I sat there, nearly dropping, suddenly I heard a popping,
A very distinct, alarming popping, that I hadn't heard
     a moment before.
"Just a bottle cap," I muttered,
"only this and nothing more,"

Ah distinctly I remember, it was in the bleak December,
One of the months I'd bought my rollers for.
But, for whatever reason — probably fear of next year's
     racing season —
A real ride had sounded pleasing, so I grabbed my bike and
     headed out the door,
Never suspecting what lay in store.

Reluctantly I glanced at my rear tire, to discover what
     had just transpired,
And I found the situation dire: It was flatter than a board.
When it comes to bike repair, I'm a failure; I don't know my ass
     from a rear derailleur.
So I started swearing like a sailor, praying for a bicycle store . . .
Surely there would be a bicycle store.

But there was nothing around except trees and cattle. Wearily, I
     climbed out of the saddle,
With aching legs and a bad case of saddle sore.
I remember thinking it would be quite a drag, if there was
     nothing useful in my saddle bag.
There had in fact been quite a lag since last I'd checked
     it, months before.
Sure enough, I found some tire levers and half a Powerbar.
Only this and nothing more.

Eagerly I sought the morrow, vainly I wished I thought to borrow
A spare tube from the guy next door.
It was slowly getting colder, and the day was growing older,

It was all too much to shoulder. I just didn't want to be
    out there anymore.
I'm really not all that hardcore.

So there I sat, on my sore ischial tuberosities, pondering all
    of these atrocities,
When suddenly a giant Raven landed on my aerobar.
And in its beak — call me a liar — was the tube I needed
    for my tire!
Now finally I could aspire to getting back to where I was before,
Before I was frozen to the core.

Quickly though I began to despair; I still had a flat
    that needed repair,
And I had never been much good at it before.
I removed the wheel with surprising ease — thank God for the
    quick release —
But the tire itself was an ordeal. With frozen fingers
    devoid of feel,
And frigid rubber inside ice-cold steel, prying it off was
    an impossible chore.
That's when the Raven said: "Nevermore"

Now I don't mean to sound sarcastic, but why are tire "irons"
    made of plastic?
The darn things kept bending like elastic. Soon my three levers
    turned to four,
When one of them snapped in half on a spoke. To the Raven this
    seemed like one big joke.
In me, violent rage did it provoke, which only got worse when it
    began to snow.
Quoth the Raven: "Nevermore."

Finally, after much consternation, and nearly digital amputation,
I felt momentary exultation as the tire slipped off and fell
    to the floor.
But then, just as quickly, I reached my nadir: My pump was
    Presta, the tube was Schrader!
And in my now demented state I could hear the Raven cackle:
"Dude. . . Nevermore!"

Chapter 6

Run

The Ins and Outs of Running

The longer I live among the humans, the less I seem to understand them. For many years, I worked in a little office tucked away in the beautiful New England countryside. The building was surrounded by running trails that climbed hillsides and curled around gorgeous ponds. And yet the treadmills in the company gym were booked solid three days in advance. You could go out for a run on a beautiful sunny day and not see a soul, and when you got back to the office the gym would be packed and there'd be a waiting list for the elliptical trainer. And these are people who work together all day long, and basically can't stand each other.

Personally, I will do anything to avoid the miserable drudgery of the treadmill. I can remember one particular wintery New England day. The windchill was something like 20 below. When I got to the locker room to change for my run, I realized that I didn't have any tights or sweatpants, just a pair of shorts. For some reason, packing a gym bag in the morning is an extremely taxing mental challenge for me. As I'm leaving the house in the morning, I'll have a vague anxiety that I've forgotten something. I'll rack my brain but I just can't imagine what it might be. And then I'll get to the locker room at lunch and I'll realize: "Oh yeah. PANTS."

But I didn't even consider the treadmill; I still had to run outside. It took only a few seconds to realize this was a major mistake. My thighs turned bright pink, and it started to feel like a scene from *Into Thin Air*. I thought about calling my family to tell them I loved them. These are the lengths I will go to avoid The Mill.

One of the many things I don't understand about treadmills is why they insist on announcing your speed in miles per hour, which is pretty much meaningless to a runner, instead of minutes per mile. Someone really needs to inform the treadmill manufacturers that "miles per hour" is relevant to motorized vehicles and maybe baseball pitchers. It's meaningless to a runner. Then again, at least I understand what a "mile per hour" is. I have absolutely no idea what a "MET" is. All I know is the treadmill seems to think it's really important.

Whenever they show pictures of those old medieval torture chambers, I always expect to see a treadmill hovering menacingly in the corner. With, of course, a medieval TV hanging from the ceiling in front of it. Those TVs don't do much to reduce the monotony for me, because if I take my eyes off my feet for more than half a second, I will lose my equilibrium and get hurtled into the floor-to-ceiling mirror at about 8.2 miles per hour — which might be the only useful reason for having the display in MPH, so you can tell the paramedic the speed you were traveling when your face hit the mirror.

One of the few good things about treadmills is that they allow you to have meaningless philosophical debates about whether running on a treadmill is an exact simulation of running real life — in other words, whether running in place with the ground moving underneath you is identical, physiologically, to running forward with the ground standing still beneath you. I'm not sure, and I don't really care, but I do know that the sensation I get for the first few seconds after I get off a treadmill is identical, physiologically, to the sensation I get after three shots of Jagermeister.

The Emperor's New Shoes

Looking for a new pair of running shoes these days is like shopping for a tropical fish — there's such a bizarre array of exotic colors and fantastic shapes. I remember when I was a kid, there were basically two kinds of footwear: regular shoes and "tennis" shoes. All the tennis shoes were made by a company called "Keds," and they all looked the same. They were all made out of white canvas, or, if the manufacturers were feeling especially wacky, blue canvas. "Keds" did not have a patented cushioning technology; you were lucky if they came with laces.

Don't get me wrong, I'm all for innovation, but buying a shoe today requires more research than buying a commercial aircraft. And about as much money. You have to know the exact chemical formula of the surface you're most likely to run on, and you need a detailed physiological analysis of your running stride to figure out whether you pronate, supinate, hibernate or whatever. Forty years ago, Steve Prefontaine managed to run pretty well in shoes made on a waffle iron in Bill Bowerman's garage. Today, shoe companies spend more on R&D than NASA, and we don't have an American runner who could hang with Pre on a beer run.

It really makes you wonder what's going on behind the scenes at the big shoe companies, where the products just keep getting more outlandish by the day, and they keep on pushing the envelope. (That's an expression I've never really understood, by the way. I mean, how hard is it to push an envelope?) I imagine the product development meetings probably go something like this:

> *Shoe company executive:* "All right, people, it's been several hours since the latest revolution in running shoe technology. I mean, people out there still feel comfortable running in shoes they bought last week, for heaven's sake. What have you got for me?"
>
> *First researcher:* "Well, sir, we've observed that running shoes have traditionally laced up at or near the top of the foot. How about a shoe that laces up on the bottom?"

Shoe company executive: "I like it! I always thought those laces were an eyesore. And it'll leave more room for our logo."

Second researcher: "But . . . won't it hurt to run with a bunch of laces on the bottom of your feet?"

Shoe company executive (reaching for a button under his desk): "Nonsense, feet will adapt! You must be new here. Remember who you work for, son. We are part of the biological process. Evolution will work around us."

Second researcher (hurtling out of the room though a trap door): "Aaaaaaagggghh!"

Shoe company executive: "Okay, what else have we got?"

Third researcher (with some trepidation): "Um, well, sir, in the past running shoes have all been made out of a solid material of some kind."

Shoe company executive: "I'm with you. So, where do we go from here?"

Third researcher: "Well, we've consulted with the physicists, and we see two promising options: liquid and gas."

Shoe company executive: "Liquid running shoes? I love it! Maybe that'll stop all the darn whining about blisters. Let's get going on that, I want a prototype in my office by Friday. Okay, now we're rolling. What else?"

Fourth researcher: "Well, why stop there? Another thing that's always been true about running shoes in the past is that they all actually. . . exist."

Shoe company executive: "Talk to me, baby!"

Fourth researcher: "Well, why not develop a new model of running shoe that is purely. . . theoretical."

Shoe company executive: "By god, that's brilliant! High in concept, very low in overhead. We just might be able to pull it off. But we'd need the perfect name."

Fourth researcher: "That's easy. Check this out: The Air Emperor. Get it?"

Shoe company executive: "Perfect! Hey, if you can mock consumers while taking their money, all the better. Quick, someone get this researcher a couple million stock options."

Fourth researcher: "Yesss!"

Shoe company executive: "Wait a minute! Are you out of your mind? This is out of the question!"

Fourth researcher (alarmed): "What do you mean? Why?"

Shoe company executive: "Where the heck will we put the logo?"

Fourth researcher: "Oh my god! I forgot about that. Does this mean I'm not gonna get those stock op . . . Aaaaaaaaggghh!"

Ticked Off About Time

It turns out that the hardest thing about triathlon isn't the constant training, it isn't trying to balance the demands of the sport with work and family, it isn't having to do five times as much laundry as a normal person. It isn't even trying to open the wrapper on a PowerBar with your teeth during a bike ride.

Nope, it turns out that the hardest part of triathlon, by far, is the math. My body can handle the physical pounding, but the constant, grueling computations are wearing me down.

Let's say I go out for a training run that takes me 45:24, according to my extremely precise training watch, plus the 30 additional seconds it took me to remember to start the damn thing at the beginning of the run, minus the 15 seconds it took me to stop and tie my shoelaces. According to my rough calculations, that yields a net elapsed time of 45:39. That's the easy part. Now suppose I know that the course I ran is 5.5 miles long. I know this because I measured it on my extremely precise bike computer, which I was able to program only after completing the series of computations set out in the technical manual, which involved, among other things, the circumference and diameter of my wheels, the length of my inseam, the value of Pi, and the speed of the earth's rotation.

Anyway, if I wanted to figure out what pace I was running, it would take me all afternoon, a notebook full of scratch paper and a slide rule. The root of the problem, in my opinion, is time. Time is all screwed up. I would like to get my hands on the genius who decided that, even though the rest of the world was happily operating under the "Base 10" system in which everything goes up to 100 and then starts over at 1, time, for some reason, can only go up to 60.

If time worked like everything else, then 45 minutes and 39 seconds would work out to 45.39 minutes, and it would be a relatively manageable project to divide by the distance and figure out my pace. But noooooooo, they had to get cute and stop counting seconds at 60 instead of 100, which means that first you've got to figure out what fraction of a minute :39 represents, which involves dividing 39 by 60, and then, after dividing the time by 5.5 miles, you have to convert the number back into the Base 60 system to figure out your actual pace.

That's a whole lot of effort for a brain already operating with minimal oxygen intake. If you ever have to perform these calculations under actual race conditions, you can pretty much forget it. I remember one race when I was trying to break 40 minutes in a tough 10k. When I got to the 4-mile marker, my watch said 26:14. Trying to figure out what pace I had to run the rest of the way nearly made my head explode. First, I had to figure out how much time was left between 26:14 and 40:00, which involves *subtracting* time, no picnic in itself, and then I had to convert the seconds into minutes and then try to divide by the 2.2 miles left in the race. After a lot of mental exertion, I decided I'd better just run as fast as I darn could, and left it at that.

You'd think technology would be a big help in all of this, but no such luck. My training watch, although extremely competent at telling me how much time has elapsed, isn't a whole lot of help with much else, unless some of those buttons do a lot more than I think they do, which is entirely possible since I don't know what half of them do in the first place. I'm convinced someone sneaks into my room at night and switches all of them around, because the "start/stop" button has never been in the same spot on my watch for two consecutive runs.

Weather Advisory

As triathletes, we've all gotten used to getting mocked on a pretty regular basis. We get mocked by schoolchildren yelling "Go faster!" out the window of their school buses as they pass us on our bikes. We get mocked by the locals in the towns we race in on Sunday mornings, who look at us incredulously through the dirty windows of Dunkin' Donuts at 6 a.m. as if we'd just landed from another planet. We even get mocked by our own loved ones, who sometimes find our behavior a little eccentric (seriously, is it really all that crazy to run the five miles from a wedding ceremony to the reception in order to squeeze in a workout?).

But I think it's fair to say that nothing mocks us as regularly, or as effectively, as the Weather. The Weather takes it as a personal insult when we try to plan a workout without taking it into account, and it will do everything in its power to make us pay the price. This is why, if your schedule calls for a hard bike ride on Wednesday before work, the Weather will see to it that Wednesday dawns with a sky right out of a Van Gogh painting, with swirling winds, freezing temperatures and hailstones the size of freewheels. And then, of course, when 10 a.m. rolls around, and you look past your bottle of Comtrex out your office window, you see nothing but blue sky and sunshine — and you can almost hear the Weather chuckling in the distance.

We do, however, have some limited ability to control the Weather. For example, on those rare bike rides when we actually think to pack our rain gear, this pretty much guarantees that it will be dry as a desert all day long. But if we don't, then even if it's a perfectly clear day and we're only riding three miles down the street to the bagel shop, a thunderclap will materialize out of nowhere right over our heads. Those ancient civilizations that tried to end droughts by doing that silly Rain Dance were wasting their time. All they needed to do was head out for a century ride and forget to pack their rain gear.

Sometimes, though, we have only ourselves to blame for our Weather-related misfortunes. For example, I don't know about you, but this is how I determine how cold it is outside before heading out for a run: I look out the window. As if I can tell 30 degrees and sunny from 60 degrees and sunny just by looking at it. I'm much too lazy to waste the 15 seconds it would take to check the weather online.

And it's not as if I'm usually right. In fact, the evidence strongly suggests that I have no weather detection skills whatsoever. I'll leave the house in shorts and a T-shirt, and within seconds the wind chill will turn my exposed skin the color of raw salmon. Of course, even though I'm only 50 yards from my front door, it's way too late to go back home and change, because you can't let the Weather win. So I suffer through it.

Then, the very next morning, it'll look pretty much the same out the window, and so I'll think to myself that I'm not going to make *that* mistake again, and I'll dress like I'm heading out on the Iditarod. And of course it'll be 85 degrees, and I'll have to shed layers every quarter-mile like some kind of bizarre and not particularly sexy aerobic striptease, and then drive the course afterward to retrieve all the articles of clothing I've hidden in bushes and under rocks.

I suppose it's possible that this is all an elaborate subconscious plot to create an excuse for dogging it in my workout. Because we all know that the intensity of a workout is inversely proportional to the nastiness of the weather. In other words, if you've forced yourself to get outside for a run in some truly horrendous weather, you get "workout points" for that effort, which you can then use to downgrade the intensity of your run. So, for example, a three-mile run at a leisurely pace in a driving rainstorm is equivalent to a five-mile interval run on a beautiful sunny day. This is a mode of thinking that sports-weather psychologists refer to as "meteorillogical reasoning." Or they would, if there were such a thing as sports-weather psychologists. Which, clearly, there should be.

Getting Lost

You might have noticed a rash of highly publicized incidents lately involving athletes getting lost on race courses during triathlons. It's hard to understand exactly how this happens. Even though we like to talk about all the thought and strategy that goes on during the race, let's be honest — there really isn't a whole lot to think about most of the time. Basically, all you've got to concentrate on is (1) what body part hurts the most right now, and (2) what direction you're supposed to go next. I don't want to antagonize those of you who have had an off-course experience (the politically correct phrase for getting lost), but this doesn't seem like an overly taxing mental challenge.

It's particularly odd because most triathletes are somewhat anal-retentive to begin with, and so terrified of getting lost during a race they become maniacally obsessed with making sure they're going in the right direction at all times. I've served as a course marshal and can attest to this from personal experience. You could have a giant, twenty-foot-tall flashing neon arrow at an intersection pointing in the right direction, and hysterical athletes will still scream "WHICH WAY??!!" at the marshals as they approach the corner.

All of which makes the increased frequency of lost triathletes extremely mysterious. Are race courses getting more complex? Are race marshals getting more lackadaisical? Or are we triathletes just getting plain stupider? The answers are unclear. But what is clear is that getting lost during a race is the triathlon equivalent of slipping on a banana peel. It can be highly amusing. . . provided, of course, it's not happening to you.

It usually starts with a general feeling of uneasiness that you can't quite put your finger on. You're racing along, minding your own business, when it slowly dawns on you that there's no one else around. This seems strange. Could the pack really be that spread out? You start looking over your shoulder, hoping to catch a glimpse of a bike or a runner. Your brain is desperate to avoid the conclusion that you've gone off course, because the consequences, physical and psychological, are just too brutal. It's like those nightmares you had as a kid, the ones where you stayed up all night studying for the wrong exam. So you convince yourself that the next arrow is just around the bend.

But with each passing second, grim reality starts to set in, and that knot starts growing bigger in the pit of your stomach. At some point, you've got to accept the fact that you're lost and start retracing your steps. But when? How do you know when it's time to give up, curse as loudly and obscenely as you can, and turn back in the other direction? It's even worse when a pack of triathletes gets lost as a group. Because then everyone assumes that everyone else knows where they're going, and the whole pack just keeps cruising off course like an electron spun off in a chain reaction.

Once the race is over, two things usually happen. First, you get to have some fun crunching the numbers, convincing yourself that if not for the miscue, you not only would have set a PR, but also shaved 10 minutes off the course record. It's amazing how many triathletes have career races on days when they happened to get lost. Second, you immediately start looking for someone to blame. The course marshals are an obvious target. I will admit that sometimes course marshals can be a little casual when it comes to giving directions — as if, just by standing motionless at an intersection, athletes speeding by at 30 miles per hour will be able to tell from their body language or facial expression which direction to go.

But the truth is, given the relatively small percentage of athletes who manage to get lost during an event, statistically the responsibility probably has to fall on the athletes themselves. It is well documented that triathletes can suffer from major lapses in concentration. Often, these occur during the pre-race instructions. Does anyone actually listen to the instructions anymore? The race director will spend twenty minutes yelling into a bullhorn about the five waves at the swim start, and inevitably a competitor who had been preoccupied trying to fasten the Velcro on the back of his wetsuit will raise his hand and ask, "Are there going to be waves, or is it mass start?" With that kind of focus, it's not hard to imagine missing an arrow or two out on the course.

Chapter 7

Race Day

Just Warming Up

Warming up before a race is absolutely critical to achieving peak performance. I know this because I have never warmed up properly before a race . . . and I have never had a peak performance.

Race after race, it's always the same story for me. The day before every event I promise myself that this time it's gonna be different. I'm gonna eat an appropriate pre-race meal, get to sleep at a reasonable hour, get to the race extra early, go through a nice leisurely warm-up in all three events, and then have MY BEST RACE EVER . . .

But something always goes wrong. Next thing I know, it's fifteen minutes before the start, and I'm careening down the highway at 80 miles an hour, burping up the cheeseburger I ate at 1:00 in the morning, checking the directions to the race site with one eye while making sure my bike hasn't fallen off the rack with the other. Ever tried getting into a wetsuit while doing 80 on the highway? It's hard enough standing on the beach slathered in Vaseline. It's gotten to the point where I consider it a successful warm-up if I can find a reasonably clean bathroom with toilet paper and a door that closes — and that's just in my apartment.

Of course, even when I do manage to show up at a reasonable time before the start, it still doesn't seem to do me any good. This is due to a well-established phenomenon in which as much as 45 minutes of actual time are known to mysteriously disappear without explanation on race-day mornings. There is some kind of hiccup in the space-time continuum that happens in the moments before the start of a tri. I don't know whether I suffer from blackouts or what, but I would swear in an affidavit that there have been many race mornings when my watch has gone directly from 7:15 to 8:01. One minute I'm earnestly safety-pinning my race number to my shirt — and frequently to several layers of skin as well — thinking I've got plenty of time to spare. The next minute I notice it's gotten awfully quiet in the transition area, and I look up to find everyone knee-deep in the water. Of course, this "missing time" is fully compensated for immediately after the gun, when the next hour-and-a-half feels like it lasts approximately three days.

There's one thing in particular about warm-ups, though, that really drives me nuts. Every single race morning, for as long as I can remember — which admittedly isn't that long — as I'm driving frantically to the race, I always pass the same people out on their bikes, casually going about their warm-up rides. Can someone please tell me: Who are these people?? Don't they sleep? I mean, I'm seeing these people 10 or 20 miles from the transition area! They're getting in more mileage before the race than I rack up in a week. One day I'm going to have to ask one of these maniacs how they do it. They're easy to find: They're all up on the podium during the awards presentation.

The P.O.G.

OK, let me apologize in advance for the blatant sexism of this chapter. I generally think of myself as a pretty progressive, nonjudgmental guy in these kinds of areas. But I hope you'll agree that, in this one instance, a little gender stereotyping is totally appropriate.

Before I go on, in a lame and obvious attempt to "reach out" to all the female readers of this book, let me offer this irrelevant but perfectly honest observation: On a normal day, when I go out for a run, it usually seems to me that the makeup of the other runners I encounter, gender-wise, is more or less 50-50. But when the weather turns nasty, when it's one of those swirling, windy, wet days when the rain feels like pins and needles stinging you in the face, I swear all of a sudden it seems like 90 percent of the runners are women. It's like all the men suddenly decided it's time for a rest day, and stayed home watching golf on TV.

OK, now that this pathetic olive branch has been extended, let's get to the point. I think this is a subject that will be absolutely familiar to anyone who has ever attended a triathlon at any time in his or her life. It is a sight we have all seen countless times, a sight that is now as familiar as rows of aluminum bike racks and orange buoys floating in a misty pond.

I am referring, of course, to the Pissed-Off Girlfriend.

There has been at least one P.O.G. at every triathlon I have ever attended, and probably every triathlon that has ever been staged — in fact, I think it is now a USA Triathlon requirement. They always look exactly the same: hair a mess, eyes puffy and red, shivering, arms crossed, wearing a sweatshirt twelve sizes too big, and bearing a facial expression of utter hostility that screams, "What in the world am I doing out here at 6 a.m. on a Sunday morning watching all these losers run around in their underwear?"

Some of you are probably thinking there are just as many Pissed-Off Boyfriends at races, and maybe this is true. Maybe I just don't notice them because of my own personal biases. But I'm skeptical. I realize I am treading into deeper and deeper water here, but my guess is that going to watch your girlfriend compete in a triathlon is just a little bit too much of a blow to the ego for most guys. Of course, I'm not defending this behavior. Guys should be secure enough to handle this kind of thing. I'm just saying that it's a bit like a guy asking his wife to come to the hospital to watch him give birth to their first child.

I read an article once in which behavioral psychiatrists claimed that they can predict how long a relationship is likely to last by observing a couple having an argument. I think a triathlon might be an even better litmus test. You can pretty much predict the fate of a relationship by observing the P.O.G. during a race. If she's out at the three-mile marker handing out cups of Gatorade, things are looking good. On the other hand, if she's at Starbucks having a latte before the swimmers hit the first buoy, this means trouble.

Bad Race? Blame it on Shrdlu.

My wise old training partner Jim Murphy used to say: "If something can go wrong, it will go wrong . . . but only during a race, never during training." This, of course, was before he was eaten by a giant squid during the Third Annual Sea Carnivore Triathlon off the coast of Australia last summer. You might have heard about it.

Murphy's law has been proven time and again. A statistically unnatural number of things always seem to go wrong during competition — when they can cause complete disaster, cost you lots of money, wreck your racing schedule and make you look like a total fool in front of the entire racing community — rather than during training, when they wouldn't really be that big a deal.

Printers have come up with a plausible explanation for this phenomenon: Shrdlu. According to printing legend, Shrdlu is the invisible Gremlin who sneaks into the press room late at night, after everything has been proofed 1000 times, and entertains himself by switching the captions under the photos of the local candidate for Mayor and the latest convicted felon, inserting embarrassing headlines such as "Local Marathoner Beaten by Foot," and generally making a total mess of things.

My theory is that Shrdlu has taken up triathlon, and now spends a lot of his spare time hanging around transition areas, messing with everyone's gear. How else do you explain, for example, bike computers? Let's say I put in an average of 250 training miles a week (I don't come close, but let's say I do — that's the beauty of writing), and that I average maybe 50 racing miles per month, and only in the summer. This means that the probability of the battery in my computer dying during a race, as opposed to during a training ride, is roughly 1 in . . . um . . . well, let's just say it's not very high.

Completely fabricated empirical data, however, has proven that bike computers are 10,000 times more likely to go on the fritz during a race than on a training ride. (By the way, where does the expression "on the fritz" come from? Was there someone named Fritz whose stuff never worked right? And did he know my friend Jim Murphy?) It's a well-known fact that computer batteries will sit back and wait patiently for your next race, reliably ticking out RPMs and tenths of miles. As soon as you strip off your wetsuit and head out of the parking lot, the computer will start flashing bizarre, demonic messages at you before announcing that you're currently cruising at 88.88 mph. You can almost hear Shrdlu chuckling in the background.

And that's only one example. Flat tires, shoelaces and excruciatingly painful race-day blisters all operate on the same basic principle. No one is safe from Shrdlu, but it has become clear to me that I've become a special project of his. Take the following absolutely true account of one particularly memorable race last summer. A buddy had flown in from Chicago to do a Sunday-morning race about an hour outside of town, requiring us to wake up at a preposterously early hour — the kind of time you'd never actually experience with an "a.m" after the number, except for these darn races. Because we are responsible, committed triathletes, we made sure we got to bed a solid 45 minutes before the wake-up call. Somehow, we managed to get up at the appointed time, grab what we hoped was our gear and stumble out to the car.

But Shrdlu was waiting for us. I tried starting the car, but the battery was deader than our brain cells. Clearly, Shrdlu has infiltrated the entire battery community, both car and computer. At first, I thought it was no big deal. A friend who was doing the race lived nearby. All we had to do was give him a call and mooch a ride. I tried his cell phone. No answer. Sent him a text — ALL CAPS, with multiple exclamation points. No response. Shrdlu had thought of this. I learned later that in his race-morning haze my friend had forgotten to grab his cell phone.

Now we were in serious trouble. At that point, I figured there's only one thing left to do. I knew that some local triathletes usually met on race mornings in front of a health club about five miles from my place. Our only hope was to bike down there as hard as we could — the ultimate time trial — and try to catch them before they took off.

So there we were, cranking at race pace down the highway into town at 5:00 on a Sunday morning. There were no water stations. I felt like a character in a Road Runner cartoon. In fact, the whole episode had become completely surreal, and I wasn't entirely sure if it was actually happening or if it was a nightmare. I was rooting hard for the nightmare.

As we rounded the last turn and headed toward the meeting spot, I was sure everyone would still be there. We were barely late and this group hadn't left on schedule in the entire history of recorded time. But Shrdlu had seen to it that we'd arrive moments after they left. Defeated, we started our cool-down ride back home. But then I had one last, desperate idea. I got out my cell phone and dialed AAA. Naturally, my membership had just expired, so they had to transfer me to New Accounts to re-enlist for another year. Then — finally! — we caught a break. The AAA rep on the phone was a runner and instantly understood the gravity of the situation. He promised to have a truck there as soon as possible. Good thing we weren't a family of five stuck on the side of the road in a snowstorm!

We pulled back into my driveway and the tow truck pulled in seconds later. Finally things were starting to go our way. The mechanic got my car going, and we drove like lunatics to the race. We got to the registration table with moments to spare, and I was feeling triumphant — until I unpacked my gear bag.

Luckily, someone had an extra pair of goggles to lend me. Nice try, Shrdlu.

Deja Vu

The morning had a very familiar feeling to it. My alarm went off at the usual grotesquely early hour, and I awoke with that familiar feeling of anticipation mixed with dread. I struggled out of bed, wondering how I'd gotten myself into this. I knew it was a bad idea to eat a lot before an event like this, but I was starving, so I guiltily ate half a granola bar. Then I grabbed the bag of gear I'd packed the night before, and headed out into the still-dark morning, knowing I was in for some serious suffering.

Unfortunately, my destination wasn't some bucolic pond for the start of a sprint triathlon. It was John Dempsey Hospital in Farmington, Connecticut, where I had pre-registered for an appointment with a surgeon to repair the Achilles tendon I'd torn a couple days before. But I felt right at home, because the similarities to race day were uncanny.

When I arrived at the site, there was the usual long line at the registration table. Finally, I got to the check-in counter. When I signed in, they assigned me a number and handed me a bag of stuff, most of it useless. Instead of a T-shirt, I got a hospital gown. At least I didn't already have a drawer full of those. There seemed to be a lot of chaos, people running around all over the place trying to get ready. A friend even offered to come along to show support, and ended up handing me little cups of water all morning long. The sense of deja vu was overwhelming.

As usual, I was shocked when I saw the registration fee — just like triathlon entry fees, health care costs are spiraling out of control. But at least this time, I didn't have to regret not signing up for early registration. And there was no one-day USAT membership fee. Plus, ninety percent was paid by insurance, which gave me a really good idea for a new business: Entry fee insurance. We just need to find some triathlete actuaries to figure out what kind of people are most likely to get injured or lazy (or, in my case, both) and blow off races, and calculate premiums accordingly. We'll make a fortune. Although I have a sneaking suspicion I might wind up in the highest risk category.

So anyway, after registration, we were sent off to the staging area, where I had to get undressed in front of a bunch of total strangers — again, something I was pretty comfortable with. A body marker came by to write on my leg, just like on race day.

Then someone else came by and actually shaved my leg for me, which I thought was a really nice touch. I asked her to do both legs while she was at it, but she declined.

Then it was time for the pre-event instructions. Like always, I was so geared up to get on with it that I didn't pay much attention. I figured if they had anything really important to tell me, they would have told me by now. Finally, it was time to get started. As usual, after all the anxiety and preparation, the event itself was anticlimactic. I don't remember much of it. But I do have one suggestion: Forget all the water stations and bike mechanics and clothing expos and that other stuff. All USAT-sanctioned events really ought to have an anesthesiologist stationed in the transition area.

After it was over, I was in some pain for a while and felt like puking, but after a fistful of ibuprofen I started feeling better. I was eager to get the results, but as usual they took forever. Finally, I went home, exhausted, and spent the rest of the weekend lying on the couch watching TV. Only this time, instead of taking the next day off from training, I had an excuse for the next three months.

It's All Relative

As triathletes, I'm sure you all share my grave concern about the Theory of Relativity. Here's my issue: As I understand it — and you triathlete-physicists out there can correct me if I'm wrong — the Theory of Relativity holds that time and speed are relative, and that time actually slows down when objects begin traveling at faster speeds.

Well, if that's true, then it's no wonder faster triathletes have been kicking my butt to the finish line all these years — they've got a hell of a lot more time to get there than I do! If you ask me, that's an unfair advantage. And I see only two ways of eliminating it. One would be to require all triathletes to travel at exactly the same speed, which would certainly make for some very dramatic finishes. The second would be to push the finish line proportionally farther back, depending on how fast people are going, to balance out the time factor. Either one would be OK with me, and would make the sport a whole lot fairer and allow all of us to compete on a "level playing field."

While we're at it, I would also like to discuss a closely related concept, the Theory of Relativity of Pain, which is a very familiar principle to all triathletes. The Theory of Relativity of Pain holds that incidents that would cause most of us to collapse in tears if they happened on an ordinary day — such as having a rock the size of a small rodent wedged inside your running shoe — somehow go completely unnoticed during a triathlon, when they have to compete for attention with other pressing matters, such as your lungs straining to take in enough oxygen to keep your major organs from shutting down.

I'm convinced that I could have several fingers bitten off during the swim by a competitor or a vicious sea creature (and what's the difference, really?), and I wouldn't notice until after the race when I'm trying to open the wrapper on an energy bar, which is damn hard enough with all ten fingers. The medical profession could sharply reduce costs by doing away with anesthesia and conducting all surgical procedures during triathlons. I think I'm going to ask my dentist if he'd mind doing my next cleaning in the transition area early one Sunday morning.

Which Way to the Race?

Cartography — the science of map-making — has made tremendous strides over the past several centuries. Maps, which used to consist of little more than rough outlines of continents and fire-breathing dragons, now convey all sorts of detailed and vital topographic information about highway systems, political boundaries and the locations of rental car companies.

Unfortunately, triathletes seem to have been left behind by these advances, like isolated tropical islands that missed out on the development of electricity and running water. If you want to get a handle on the current state of triathlon-related map-making, you wouldn't have to look much further than the pre-race information kit — you know, the packet of material that's supposed to arrive before the race, but generally arrives in your mailbox several days after the race results are posted.

One of the most important items in the pre-race kit is the directions to the race. Based on their years of experience, race directors have learned that one of the critical elements of staging a successful race is making sure that people know where the race is actually being held. Because races are usually held in remote, obscure public parks that are more or less "off the grid," MapQuest is not usually all that much help, making directions all the more critical. Unfortunately, the map in the pre-race kit generally consists of an enlargement of a page from a world atlas, with some helpful notes scribbled in the margin. If the race were being held in, say, Rhode Island, a typical map would depict the entire mid-Atlantic region of the United States, with a little arrow floating out in the Atlantic next to the hand-written notation, "RACE."

The imprecision of these directions lends an additional element of adventure to the already challenging race-morning routine. Usually, you have a vague recollection of the directions because you raced the same course three or four years ago. But, because the race areas all look so similar, and because it's 5:15 in the morning, and because your brain is already stressing over such issues as whether you remembered to pack your bike helmet, your memory is never quite sharp enough to remember whether you're supposed to turn right or left at the Dunkin' Donuts. The race directors try to help out by posting amusing but not particularly helpful signs to guide you along the way. On one recent race-morning drive, we encountered signs posted at critical inter-sections along the way that looked — I am not making this up — exactly like this:

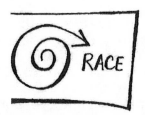

Luckily, though, once you get close it's fairly easy to find your way to the race by drafting off the back of the first SUV you see with three tri-bikes mounted on the roof. Since it's before dawn on a Sunday morning, unless there is an early Mass at the Church of the Latter Day Cyclists, it's a pretty safe bet that the SUV is heading to the race. Before long, you'll have a whole caravan of cars with bikes strapped to their roofs, looking like the bizarre skeleton of a Stegosaurus winding its way down the road (and, given my age group, dinosaurs are an apt analogy). Usually, though, just when you think you're finally heading the right way and the race must be right around the bend, you pass a Stegosaurus whizzing by in the other direction. The only question at that point is which Stegosaurus is heading the right way, and which is heading toward extinction.

Web of Despair

There has been a lot of debate over the past few years about whether the Internet, with its nearly instantaneous distribution of news and information, has had a positive or negative overall effect on our quality of life. While the jury is still out on that larger issue, I think we can all agree that there is one area in which the Internet has completely revolutionized the distribution of information. I refer, of course, to online race results. Race directors can now get results posted with impressive speed. In many cases, by the time you drive home from the race and shower, you can already log in and see just how many competitors in their 70s and 80s finished ahead of you.

You could, that is, if you had any idea where to look. I don't know about you, but I've spent hours of frustration trying to find race results tucked away in some remote corner of the Web. Let's say you just finished a race called Joe's Triathlon. You'd think all you have to do is go to www.joestriathlon.com, where you'd find a giant flashing link in the center of the screen saying "CLICK HERE FOR RACE RESULTS!" I mean, why else would I be logging into the website after the race is already over?

But life isn't that simple. The problem is, usually it isn't Joe who's posting the results. Joe is just a regular guy with a day job who decided to organize a triathlon in his spare time just to further alienate himself from his family and friends, and quite frankly, putting the race together was such a pain in the ass that now that it's over with, he's pretty much done thinking about it for a while, thank you very much. Instead, the results are posted by the companies that do the timing for the race, so they usually end up on websites with such obvious and intuitive URLs as www.industrialtimingsystems.com/triathlon/october/2011/joes/howintheworlddidufindthissite?

Even if you're lucky enough to find the right website, you're still not out of the digital woods. The next problem you face is that the typical computer screen isn't tall enough to display all the names or wide enough to display all the columns at the same time. This means that unless your name is up at the top of the list (which I can assure you mine is generally not), you have to scroll down the page to find it, at which point you can't see the headings for the columns that tell you which numbers are which. Then, once you find your name, you have to scroll over to the right to see all your times, at which point you can no longer see the names to know which row is yours. At that point, you are looking at a screen that pretty much looks like this:

14:48	1:32	1:23:01	1:56	44:25	2:35:10
16:04	1:37	1:14:49	2:07	49:47	2:37:09
15:27	2:09	1:16:26	2:57	48:40	2:39:27
17:48	1:35	1:24:01	1:56	44:25	2:41:10
17:55	1:56	1:31:09	2:14	41:45	2:46:16

Whether these are triathlon race results or some new software code from Microsoft is anybody's guess. I don't think this is what the Internet marketing people have in mind when they talk about a "positive user experience."

Chapter 8

Idiosyncrasies

Nature Versus Nurture

Some of you might remember a hilarious movie called *Dazed and Confused*, about a group of high school kids growing up in the '70s. Every time I've seen it — I'm too embarrassed to disclose the actual number, but let's just say it's helped me through many a Computrainer workout — I'm amazed at how each of the characters vividly reminds me of someone from my own high school class.

For example, there's the stoner kid who spent hours sitting cross-legged on the hood of a car fascinated by the patterns on a $1 bill, and who was clearly modeled after my high school friend Tom. And there was the slacker ex-football player, played by Matthew McConaughey, who could never quite get past high school and was still hanging out with the local kids even though he was about a decade out of school. All I can say about this character is, there's one old high school classmate of mine that I really hope is getting rich off the royalties.

By now, you're probably wondering, OK, what if anything does this have to do with triathlon? The answer, to be perfectly honest, is not a whole lot. But it goes well beyond the absolutely true fact that my old high school friend Tom became a darn good elite triathlete when he grew up. I bet the monotony of those long training runs is a breeze for someone who can get hours of entertainment out of a dollar bill.

The real answer is that every time I move to a new city or travel to a race in some new part of the world, I have an experience that's a lot like watching *Dazed and Confused*. Without fail, the characters I run into are carbon copies of the lunatics that I race and train with back home. It's as if there's a hidden "triathlete" gene marker buried somewhere in our DNA. Maybe we can get some federal grant money to study this phenomenon. On the other hand, forget it, we'd probably just blow the cash on titanium spokes.

I first discovered the gene marker a few years back when I did a sprint triathlon in Melbourne, Australia. I expected to marvel at the cultural differences between the triathlon community back home and this one 14,000 miles away. No such thing. There it all was: the same bad '70s music, the same jovial but disorganized volunteers trying furiously to get everyone registered, the same cheesy T-shirts, the same portable bike shops set up like MASH units hawking shorts and used bike components, the same harried race director frantically yelling instructions into a bullhorn. About the only way I could tell I wasn't in Massachusetts or Connecticut was by listening to the instructions. At one point, for example, the race director announced to the group in his thick Australian accent that "you'll be going flat-out at 40k but it'll all come a cropper when you hit the roundabout." Which, I later learned, meant that there would be a nasty headwind on the second half of the bike course. Or something like that.

But the phenomenon of the triathlete gene marker was really driven home a few years ago when I moved from Boston to Connecticut. Up in Boston, I belonged to a little triathlon club that was founded at a local health club by a serene, silver-haired, 50ish Svengali-like triathlete and his training partner, a gruff Italian guy who spoke to no one, whose workouts were legendary and who terrified the other health club members when they were foolish enough to get in his way.

When I moved to Connecticut, the first thing I did was join a local health club, and sure enough, it was like stepping into a parallel universe. There was a little triathlon club run by, I am not making this up, a serene, silver-haired, 50ish Svengali-like figure. A few days later, in the pool, I encountered his training partner, who of course did not actually speak to me but who was kind enough to instruct his 9-year-old son to hang out in my lane so as not to disturb him during his workout. I am still on the lookout for a guy with a ponytail, sitting in the corner of the club, studying a $1 bill.

Risky Business?

Ok, quick quiz. See if you can identify which of the following activities doesn't belong on this list:

- Swimming

- Biking

- Running

- Careening down a raging river in a flimsy inflatable rubber raft while some spaced-out hippie screams incoherent instructions at you and your backside is repeatedly assaulted by jagged rocks and a raftload of clueless yuppies keeps whacking you in the head with plastic paddles.

Seems pretty straightforward, doesn't it? Well, that's what I thought, too, but it turned out to be a major brain-teaser to a group of friends who recently decided to organize a white-water rafting/suicide trip, and somehow decided that, since I am a tri-athlete, I'd be dying to go.

As near as I can figure, their reasoning went something like this:

- White-water rafting involves water.

- Triathlon involves water.

- Conclusion: We're desperate to find someone else foolish enough to shell out a couple hundred bucks for this trip, so who cares if this logic doesn't make a whole lot of sense?

Unfortunately, this happens all the time. For whatever reason, people seem to group triathlon with a whole range of high-risk, "adventure" sports like skydiving, white-water rafting and bungee-jumping. And let's face it, we don't go out of our way to discourage this misperception. We walk around saying "dude" a lot, sporting tattoos (many of them temporary), and trying to act rugged and fearless and carefree, like we're surfers or something. This is a total fraud, of course, because the reality is that in terms of overal carefreeness, triathletes rank just a notch or two below IRS agents.

As a group, we're about as risk-averse as you can get. What we want is control, not risk. We obsess about a race for months in advance. By the time race day rolls around, we've mapped out every conceivable detail. We lay out our gear the night before; we know exactly what we're going to eat in the morning; we monitor our liquid intake to the millimeter; we know exactly how many miles we're going to bike for our warm-up; we know exactly how many times we're going to pee before the race starts. We still manage to screw a tremendous amount of it up, of course, but that's beside the point.

Our physical well-being is where our neurotic, uptight person-alities reach their anal-retentive peak. Without exception, triath-letes are textbook hypochondriacs. We obsess over every little physiological detail of our bodies, every twinge and ache and pain. We memorize and chart our resting heart rates and VO2 maxes and anaerobic thresholds and you name it. I'm convinced that if a triathlete were to suffer a serious head injury (and I think you'll find that most of us have), he would forget his name long before his blood cholesterol level. When it comes to overall knowledge of the human cardiovascular system, I'd take a triathlete over a fourth-year med student with a copy of Gray's Anatomy.

And this is the reason you'll rarely see a triathlete bouncing around in the back of a raft heading down the rapids. This kind of activity could disrupt the triathlete's rigid control over his or her physical health. It could lead to injury, which is to a triathlete what garlic is to a vampire. An injury means you can't train, and when you can't train, you can't eat and you can't think and you can't sleep and your whole world comes crashing down around you and you have no choice except to shoot yourself in the head . . . except that this could lead to another injury.

I'm sure there's a great deal more to be said on this topic, but I'm going to stop here. I'm worried all this typing might do some-thing weird to my wrists.

One Mother of a Triathlete

Ring.

"Hello."

"Leib? Is that you?"

"Hi Mom. Yes, it's me. I'm the only one who lives here, remember?"

"I just wasn't expecting you to be home at this hour, that's all."

"Then why'd you call?"

"What, I'm not allowed to give my own son a call?"

"No, that's not what I . . . Nevermind."

"So how come you're home on a Saturday night? Shouldn't you be out with your friends? Are you sick?"

Uh oh. Looks like this might be it. The moment of truth. The moment I have to try to explain all this triathlon stuff to my Mom. This is a woman whose only concept of training also involves the word "potty." A woman whose two greatest, and perhaps only, fears are: (1) anything that poses a serious risk of harm to her children, and (2) anything that poses a non-serious risk of harm to her children.

"No Mom, I'm fine. It's just that . . . well, I have to get up really early tomorrow morning."

"Well. And what could possibly be so important to get *you* up so early on a Sunday morning?" Only a Mother — and perhaps Laurence Olivier — could tinge the simple word *you* with such a complex mix of sarcasm and . . . well, just sarcasm.

"It's sort of a . . . race."

"A race? What kind of race?"

Here we go.

"It's called a tri-ath-a-lon." I said the words slowly, so she could understand.

"Oh." Short pause. "So, what distance? Are we talking Ironman here? Olympic distance? Just a sprint? What?"

Longer pause.

"Pardon me?"

"What, you think your mother doesn't know from tri-ath-a-lon?" She was mocking me.

"Well, I . . ."

"So what distance?"

"It's just a sprint, Mom."

"You're staying in on a Saturday night just for a sprint? That's a little weak, don't you think?"

"I guess so Mom. Sorry."

"Well, since you'll be rested, might as well go out hard in the water. Don't hold anything back."

"Um . . . OK, I will, thanks."

"Got your gear all laid out?"

"Yes, Mom."

"Don't forget to . . . wait a minute, your Father's yelling something at me. He's always got to get his two cents in, your Father. What, dear? OK, OK. Your Father and I think for a sprint you should ditch the wetsuit. Costs you too much time in the transition."

"Mom, this is too weird."

"Just a suggestion. It's your life. If you don't want to listen, you don't have to listen."

"OK, I'm sorry. It's a good idea, thanks."

"So where's the tattoo?"

"*Mom?*"

"C'mon. Ankle? Calf? Shoulder? Oy vey, please don't tell me you're racing without a tattoo. Honey, you hear that? Your son is racing without a tattoo."

"But Mom, I thought you'd be upset if I —"

"You thought, you thought . . . What about looking good at the finish line, did you think about that? Where did we go wrong with you . . .?"

"Sorry, Mom."

"It's OK, it's OK. Just kick some butt tomorrow. And remember, even if you bonk on the run, your Father and I still love you very much."

There's Definitely An "I" in Triathlon

As I have pointed out before, there is a certain type of personality that is drawn to the sport of triathlon, and despite popular misconception, it is not the mellow, easygoing, golden-retriever-owning personality type. It is more the hyper-intense, neurotic, self-absorbed, OK-seriously-if-you-don't-stop-talking-about-last-night's-IM-workout-I-am-going-to-poke-my-eyeballs-out-with-this-pencil personality type.

Which is part of the reason triathlon is the ultimate individual sport. Triathletes are able to endure the endless hours of solitary training because they actually prefer listening to their own heart rates over being around anyone else — and, frankly, in most cases the feeling is pretty much mutual. Heart-rate monitor manufacturers ought to come out with a companion product called a personality monitor, which would range from a low of "mildly annoying" when the wearer has just finished a decent workout and is yammering to a colleague about her iliotibial band, to a red flashing "absolutely intolerable" when the wearer has missed two consecutive workouts due to job and family emergencies and is about to bust a blood vessel.

For this reason, triathletes generally aren't wired for "group projects" where you have to "work together" to reach "common goals." When there is a job to do, most triathletes are best left alone to work at it endlessly, by themselves, until the job is either done or, more likely, completely screwed up — in which case there'll be no one around to see it. The closest that triathlon comes to the team concept is the triathlon "relay team," but even that has been cleverly designed in such a way that each triathlete only has to be in the actual physical company of his or her teammates for a total of about a quarter of a second during the race. The rest of the time you're on your own.

This is why the whole concept of a "triathlon team" is ill-fated from the get-go. I've been on a number of these teams in different cities over the years. They just don't seem to work out all that well. Most triathletes have very firmly held opinions about the best way to get things done — often wrong, but always firmly held. When you suggest the concept of working together as a group to get something done, everyone stops and looks around in confusion and fear, like cavemen at the introduction of fire. It's a little like asking a group of elite triathletes to stop competing and run together as a pack over the final mile of a race — they're chemically unable to do it. Someone is always going to make a break for the lead. So triathlon team meetings can end up looking a lot like the famous scene in "The Godfather" where the different family Dons get together for a summit. I have been at a number of meetings like this, and I was always afraid I'd wake up the next morning and find a greasy bike wheel on the pillow next to me.

But triathlon teams are useful for one purpose — the production of the triathlon team newsletter, which has to be one of the most hilarious genres in the history of American literature. Suffice it to say that effective verbal communication is not generally the personality trait most often associated with serious triathletes, most of whom rarely express sentiments more profound than "on your left." Based on my research, it appears that there are three basic rules to putting together a triathlon newsletter: Start with a blurry photograph on the cover of an unidentifiable team member whizzing by on a bike; add creative and original news stories like "Recent Triathlon Season a Huge Success;" and finally, remember that three of virtually anything can be turned into a brilliant tri-related play on words. Seriously, how many tri-related theme parties have you been invited to in your lifetime — eat/drink/dance triathlon parties, swim/drink/bbq parties, eat/drink/passout parties. Curiously, the common denominator seems to be that drinking is always one of the legs.

Goal Oriented

To get the most out of our racing careers, most experts agree that we all need to become more goal oriented. This means that goal-setting must become an integral part of our overall training and racing strategy, right up there with calculating the optimum combination of Gu and peanut butter for your pre-race meals. Anyone can go into a racing season and just wing it, but serious triathletes will sit down long before the season starts and plot out their goals in precise and often excruciating detail. That way, they will have indisputable, documented proof of just what an abysmal failure their season was when the summer finally draws to a close.

To avoid this sense of disappointment, my advice is to set goals that are as readily achievable as possible. One useful technique is to include a number of goals that you've actually already accomplished, just to give yourself a feeling of momentum. Another tip is that, in my experience, negative goals are much easier to achieve than positive ones. "Don't attempt an Ironman-distance race under any circumstances in 2012," for example, is the kind of clear, rational, focused goal that's unlikely to come back and bite you in the rear end.

Goal-setting is a very personal, introspective process, and so it's difficult for me, an outsider, to offer much concrete guidance. However, as you begin to map out your personal goals for next year, ask yourself the following questions: What do I hope to get out of another year of racing? Am I looking to improve on last season's results or just maintain my conditioning? Was my girlfriend serious about never speaking to me again if she catches me using her razor to shave my legs in the shower?

I recently went through this intense, soul-searching process. After thoughtfully reviewing my results for the past several seasons and assessing my current physical and emotional condition, I came up with the following set of goals for next year:

- Shave 45 seconds off my 10K time

- Increase my weekly bike mileage to 250

- Finish in the top 10 percent of my age group at an Olympic-distance race

- Achieve all this without any measurable effort or sacrifice of any kind

This seemed like a pretty good effort at first. What I always recommend, though, is to walk away from your first draft for a day or two, and then come back for a reality check. When I did this, I realized that maybe these goals were a bit unrealistic, that I had to be more honest with myself or I would be set up for a huge disappointment next year. So I did the mature, responsible thing and adjusted my goals downward just a notch, finally settling on the following:

- Shave 45 seconds off my pre-race visit to the porta-potty

- Increase my annual bike mileage to 250 (including races) (and trips to the grocery store)

- Drink with people who finish in the top 10 percent of their age group at an Olympic-distance race

- Achieve all this without any measurable effort or sacrifice of any kind (hey, some things aren't negotiable!)

Now that I've gone through this difficult, painful process, I can work backward and figure out how these goals transfer into action steps for my off-season training program. I think I'll get started right away. I'm almost out of groceries.

Hunting the Wild Triathlete

I suppose it was pretty much inevitable, but my life has become an obscure cable TV show: "Leib Dodell, Triathlete Hunter."

I've moved around a lot, from D.C. to Boston to Connecticut to San Francisco to my current home in Kansas City. Each time I arrived in my new city, I became a lycra-clad anthropologist, on a mission to unearth the local triathlon community. I wanted to learn where they swam, where they did their track workouts, where they went for the cheapest all-you-can-eat buffets. So, like Charles Darwin, Jacques Cousteau and others before me, I set off on a journey into the unknown to locate and catalogue the native triathlon population.

I particularly remember my move to San Francisco. Legend had it that San Francisco was a land rich in triathletes, so I was particularly excited to get started. And it wasn't long before my trained eye picked up some telltale signs: three Treks with aero bars and Gu stickers locked in front of a GNC; two guys with shaved legs and tattoos on the subway; a sporting goods store selling nothing but wetsuits. Yep, there were triathletes here all right. Plenty of them. But after my first few weeks, I had yet to make actual contact with any of the elusive species.

I thought about setting a trap to lure some of them out into the open. It is well established in the scientific literature that tri-athletes are notoriously ravenous and cheap animals. So I figured all I had to do was put an open box of PowerBars on a park bench in the middle of the city, then hide behind a tree and wait. It was a brilliant plan, but unfortunately, I was too cheap to buy a whole box of PowerBars. And even if I had the cash, I would've been too hungry not to eat them all myself. So that idea went nowhere.

But then I had a breakthrough. Like most great scientific achievements, luck played a major tole. I was on a city bus one afternoon when I overheard two people behind me talking about going on a training ride. Suddenly, all my senses came alive. I knew this was my big chance. If this had been Mutual of Omaha's Wild Kingdom, I would've pinned one of them to the ground, clipped a homing device to his ear and released him back into the wild, so I could track them to their natural training grounds.

Luckily, that proved unnecessary. I tuned into their conversation, and sure enough they made plans to meet for a ride the next morning. I woke up early, filled with a sense of excitement and anticipation, and grabbed my bike and staked out a position near the meeting place. I waited for what seemed like an eternity. Triathlete hunting can be a lonely, solitary business. I started to worry that maybe their keen senses had picked up the presence of an outsider and scared them off.

Then, suddenly, I saw them come around a corner. There must have been a dozen of them, an entire herd of triathletes, cycling beautifully before my eyes. It unfolded in slow motion, like those scenes of giraffes galloping across the Serengeti that you see on nature shows. A chill ran up my spine as they rode by. Cautiously, I started to ride after them. I knew that packs of triathletes could be hostile to intruders. Would they accept me into their pack, or shun me as an outsider?

The triathletes were wary of me at first. Clearly, they were confused by my presence, worried that I wouldn't understand their rules and customs and cause a major pileup. But after a short time they came to realize that I meant them no harm, and they accepted me among their numbers. Like Jane Goodall and her chimpanzees, I lived among the San Francisco triathletes for the next several years. I am pleased to report that the indigenous triathlon population is healthy, thriving. . . and maybe just a little bit intense.

What's Your Hurry?

I can't believe you've actually made it this deep into the book. I can only think of two explanations for it. The first is that you're sitting on a stationary bike, or maybe stretching, or engaging in some other mind-numbingly boring activity, and the book is just a diversion to help pass the time. The second is that you're trapped somewhere, like maybe on a subway train or in a doctor's waiting room.

But one thing I'm pretty sure of is that you're not simply just sitting there, on the couch, reading this book, like a normal person. Because no triathlete in the world would have the patience for that. We are, as a class, without a doubt the single most impatient demographic group on the face of the earth. We always have to be rushing somewhere, fast, and God help anyone who gets in our way. Even if we don't have anywhere to go, we're usually in a maniacal rush to get there. Personally, I will often make myself late on purpose, just so I'll have to panic and race to get there on time.

If we're not going at maximum speed all the time, we just don't feel right. This is why racing comes so naturally to us. We do it more or less all the time anyway. This means that there are certain situations that triathletes must avoid at all costs. A triathlete in a traffic jam, for example, is not a pretty sight. You can usually spot one right away. She's the one with her head hanging out the window, Labrador-retriever-style, the veins about to burst out of her bright-red face.

The supermarket check-out line is another problem area. Again, the triathletes are easy to spot, standing in line with their shaved legs and a cart filled with pierogies and powdered sports drinks, their body language a portrait of exasperation, checking their watch more often than a track coach. Personally, I always opt for the express line — which I view as sort of the elite wave of the supermarket check-out counter — even if I have tons more shopping to do and it means I have to go through twice.

We need to recognize that this is a personality trait that makes us a bit different from the "outside world," which as general rule does not approach every moment of life with the single-mindedness and frenzied hyperactivity of the swim-bike transition. I am often reminded of being driven around by my Mom as a kid. My Mom's rate of speed ranged from stopped, which she was comfortable with in just about any weather conditions, to her top cruising speed of about 25 percent of the posted speed limit. Whenever another driver got annoyed and hurried past her, which was pretty much all the time, she would always say, with great contempt, "Well, *he* was in a big hurry." To my mother, being in a "big hurry" was just about the worst crime against humanity a person could commit. Well, I'm afraid we triathletes have become violent recidivists in the hurry department.

So what's wrong with us? I used to think it was just that we had a lot to do. Most of us train a billion hours a week, we have families to deal with, and some of us (not many, but some) even have demanding careers. So it's no wonder we're always in a hurry. We've got a lot more to do than anyone else.

But I'm afraid that's not it. Believe it or not, there are non-triathletes out there who don't spend a second training or racing, but still have very busy schedules with lots of pressing demands — albeit nothing as vitally important as a Wednesday track workout — and they manage to handle it gracefully. So I had to look elsewhere for an answer. I did a ton of research into this, and I think I've finally figured it out.

I'd love to tell you all about it, but unfortunately, I'm in an hurry and I've gotta run. . .

Mixed Marriages

I was flipping stations on the TV the other day and heard this: "Tomorrow on Jerry Springer: Triathletes and the Poor Hopeless Fools Who Love Them." OK, I didn't really hear that, but if my life is an indication, it would make for one heck of an entertaining episode.

I could probably fill the hour all by myself. I could recount, for example, the time I actually had an argument with a girlfriend — a now ex-girlfriend — while I was in the middle of a workout on my rollers. It had to be one of the more tragicomic moments in dating history. If Shakespeare had been a triathlete, this would have made a fine scene in Act III of *A Midsummer Day's Half-Ironman*. I remember the fight got worse and worse as she repeatedly asked me why I wouldn't look her in the face. I tried to explain that it was nothing personal, but if I took my eyes off my front wheel I was going to do a face-plant into the entertainment center at about 27 mph, which was definitely not part of my workout itinerary.

I have a bad feeling, though, that the vast majority of Jerry's studio audience would take her side on this. I can just picture some outraged woman waving her pocketbook at me, yelling into a hand-held microphone about why I couldn't have just stopped for one minute to have a normal conversation, and wasn't the relationship more important than my stupid workout?

The answer, of course, is no, it wasn't. I was in the middle of a set of 10 hard, two-minute intervals with a minute of spinning in between, and you can't just quit in the middle of something like that. A triathlete would understand, but there aren't likely to be too many triathletes wasting their time sitting in the studio audience for the *Jerry Springer Show*. Unless, maybe, they set up some stationary bikes.

And then I could talk about another time when — I am not making this up — I got into an argument with a girlfriend because she'd gotten hold of my training log, and was upset because I hadn't written about the dinner we'd had together the week before. I tried to explain that it was not a diary, it was a training log. There's a big difference, and there's really no combining the two. Imagine how this would sound:

Tuesday: *Killer run workout — 5 mi. warm-up on 8 min pace, six hard hill repeats, 2 mi. cooldown. Thought I'd puke my lungs out. Laurie looked beautiful in the candlelight at dinner.*

The point I'm trying to make is that sometimes it seems like triathletes and non-triathletes go together about as well as Presta and Schrader, and as far as I know, there ain't no adapter. It's kind of ironic, really. My family is always after me about dating Jewish girls — not for *their* benefit, they always say, for mine. I won't be happy unless I'm with someone who shares the same values I do, someone who I can connect with spiritually, etc. Yeah, right. If they're really concerned with my spiritual happiness, maybe they should insist I date only Jewish triathletes — an extremely small demographic. I'm pretty sure there's no dating website for that one. I think I'm doomed to wind up in one serious accident on those rollers one day.

The Long Road Back

It had been a long season and I was totally burnt out, so I decided to take a couple weeks off, just to get my edge back. Never mind that I didn't really have much of an "edge" to begin with. I still felt that a little break would help me get geared up to attack the upcoming season with new energy and enthusiasm.

But then a strange thing happened. It turned out to be kind of relaxing not to have to stress out about my workout every single day. Suddenly, I had a lot more free time. A lot fewer muscle spasms in the middle of the night. A whole lot less laundry.

Next thing I knew, those couple weeks had somehow managed to stretch into — I'm not kidding you — about 14 months. My "edge" was now buried under about 15 extra pounds of banana-nut muffins and Celeste Supreme frozen pizzas. Those muscle spasms had been replaced by spasms of guilt whenever anyone described me as a "triathlete."

So, a few weeks ago, I finally decided enough was enough. I made that critical "first step" toward getting back into serious training — I went to the store and stocked up on Advil. I figured I'd spend the first few days rebuilding my ibuprofen base. Everyone's heard of the importance of building a solid aerobic base before moving on to serious training. Well, if you've been dormant as long as I have, I figured it's also important to build a strong anesthetic base before actually attempting to head back into the gym.

Since I've now made that important first step, I thought I would pass along some other tips in case some of you out there are facing a similar predicament. The first and most important piece of advice is not to panic. This is not because your situation does not warrant panic. It does. The reason you shouldn't panic is because your cardiovascular system is in such tenuous shape, it can't take that kind of strain. You should also avoid training with other people for as long as you possibly can. People are vicious. Remember all the people in your office and your health club who pretended to be so impressed with you back when you were in racing shape? Well, secretly, they hated your guts. Like a pack of wild dogs, once they get a whiff of the fact that you're hideously out of shape, they will move in for the kill. It's tempting to think that, even after a 14-month layoff, you're still in far better shape than the average health club member laboring away on an elliptical trainer. Trust me, you're not. Beware the aerobics people in particular — they're the meanest of all. They will try to lure you innocently into the studio, telling you that a little aerobics workout will be a good steppingstone on your way back to fitness. Then, once you've wandered in there like an aging, puffy Muhammad Ali wading into the ring for his last fight, they'll pound you senseless.

My final piece of advice involves your racing bike, and my advice is simple: Leave it alone and buy a new one. My guess is that, after 14 months of dormancy, your bike is now somewhere in the corner of the garage, hosting so many exotic species of insects that federal law requires you to file an Environmental Impact Statement before giving it an overhaul. It will be far easier to go to the bike shop and buy a new one. And that capital investment will be good motivation to actually get out and ride the damn thing. But, for the first couple weeks at least, avoid those neighborhood kids riding to school on their beach cruisers. They're vicious.

Chapter 9

Ironman

A Race By Any Other Name...

Ironman. Much has been written about the drama, the pageantry, the inspirational personal stories and the brutal physical demands of this unique athletic event. Very little, however, has been written about the word "ironman" itself. This is its story.

The word "ironman" was first coined by a couple of southern California beach bums, who realized, in a moment of endorphin-induced brilliance, that if they staged a truly psychotic endurance event and came up with the perfect name for it, they could license it to the Timex Corporation for several trillion dollars.

If there was ever any doubt that they had found the perfect word, it was erased when they were immediately sued by Lou Gehrig, Cal Ripken, Jr., Marvel Comics, the heavy-metal band Black Sabbath, and John Holmes, all of whom claimed that they had been using the word "ironman" for years and had exclusive rights to it. OK, maybe that's a bit of an exaggeration. But I am not making up the fact that the World Triathlon Corporation was actually sued by Marvel Comics, on the theory that people were likely to confuse the Hawaii Ironman with their rather lame comic-book superhero "Iron Man."

This, of course, was long before Robert Downey Jr. turned Iron Man into an international film star. It was back when very few people knew who Iron Man was. He was never one of your more elite superheroes. He was more of an age-grouper, and he really didn't strike fear into the hearts of evildoers as much as amusement, because he looked like a large fire hydrant with legs. No offense to the folks at Marvel, but Iron Man *wishes* people would confuse him with the Hawaii Ironman. I bet Iron Man wouldn't even make it out of the water.

The lawsuit was ultimately settled when the WTC agreed, to minimize confusion about whether Marvel Comics was affiliated with the triathlon, that they would not allow any cartoon superheroes to actually compete in the race. I am not sure how they explain Dave Scott and Paula Newby-Fraser, but that's a problem for their lawyers.

And now I'm afraid that the second wave of triathlon litigation is about to begin, what with the Ultraman race gaining popularity. I am certain that "Ultraman," the bizarre TV-show superhero from the 1960s and 70s, is drafting his complaint as we speak.

Anyway, with "ironman" now poised to make the jump from a little-known cult term to part of the mainstream American vocabulary, now is probably the time to figure out just what, exactly, the darn word means. There seems to be a lot of confusion here. Does "ironman" refer only to races put on by the WTC — is it, in other words, the Ironman-brand Triathlon, like Band-Aid-brand adhesive strips — or does "ironman" describe any tri that goes 2.4, 112 and 26.2? I realize I am treading in some linguistically controversial waters here, but it seems to me that "ironman" ought to be in the public domain, just like "marathon."

But I don't recommend trying to stage your own "ironman" or "half-ironman" race anytime soon. The WTC's lawyers will be knocking on your door before you can put flyers under everyone's windshield wipers at the next 5k. This is too bad, because I've always thought it would be radical to stage a "Square Root of an Ironman" race, which works out to a 1.5-mile swim, 10.6-mile bike and 5.1-mile run, all perfectly plausible distances. I'm thinking, for the T-shirts, just the symbol: $\sqrt{\text{IRONMAN}}$. And don't even get me started on the Ironman^2.

Now that I think about it, if we really want to make an enduring contribution to the language, why not convert the word "ironman" into the next standard unit of distance, like the kilometer or furlong? Officially, one ironman would be equal to the combined race distance of 140.6 miles. The speed of light in a vacuum, for example, would be 1,325 ironmen per second; New York would be about 1.6 ironmen from Boston; and the circumference of the Earth would be a measly 178 ironmen. If we all work at it, this could really catch on.

But even if we can't agree on exactly what "ironman" means, I hope we can all agree that one thing it does not mean is "person who has done an ironman." I don't know about you, but I feel ridiculous referring to someone as an "ironman" — and even more ridiculous when someone uses it to refer to me. Then there is the gender problem. I have never been described as overly sensitive to these kinds of issues, but I am pretty sure that Lothar Leder would not be pleased to be described as an "ironwoman." So if we insist on "ironman" to describe the men, then in fairness we'd need a separate term for the women. For a while I was thinking maybe "iron maiden," but then of course we'd immediately get sued by the heavy-metal band.

No, the proper term for "person who has done an ironman" is simply "person who has done an ironman." If people are going to insist on a single word, then I propose "ironmaster." It is an infinitely cooler word than "ironman," it's gender neutral, and I can already see Mattel coming out with a new line of little plastic Ironmaster figurines, followed by a hugely popular Saturday-morning TV show . . . and, of course, a lot of litigation.

The Wizard of Kona

I know you're not going to believe this story, but I'm going to tell it anyway. The other day, which is when all good stories start, I was out for a bike ride, and I took a nasty little spill. I got up slowly and started pedaling again, still a little groggy.

Then a strange thing happened. A giant, twisting headwind arose from out of nowhere. My bike whirled around two or three times and then flew through the air! I sailed through the sky for what seemed like hours, until finally I landed with a thunk on a nice sandy beach. I looked around, and I could see strange looking lava fields off in the distance. Then I noticed that I was surrounded by hundreds of triathletes, all scurrying around preparing for the start of a race. And then it dawned on me. I was on the beach at Kona before the start of the Hawaii Ironman!

Except there was one weird thing. Not one of the triathletes was an inch over three feet tall! They were so small, in fact, that the numbers inked on their little arms and legs were in fractions. Very strange.

The tiny triathletes seemed really happy to see me, and they started singing and dancing around me, which I thought was a very unusual pre-race warm-up. It turned out that there had been a really wicked wind out on the course (blowing from the West, naturally), and when I flew in on my bike, somehow it died down. They were so psyched, they asked if they could do me a favor in return. I told them yes, as a matter of fact, there is something they could do. I've always dreamed of racing in Kona, but I just wasn't a strong enough runner. I'm a decent swimmer and biker. . . If I only had a run!

A buzz went through the crowd of strange little mini-triathletes and they all started whispering to each other and I didn't know what was going on. I thought maybe there was a rumor they were canceling the swim or something. Then one of them told me there was one person who might be able to help me. He was called the Wizard, and he knew all the secrets of the Ironman. He was hard to find, though, and he was kind of a jerk and might not help me even if I found him. I said as long as I was here, it was worth a try. They told me the Wizard was somewhere out on the Queen K Highway, riding the bike course.

So I started following the little yellow arrows on the road. I knew things had gotten really weird when my bike, which was now the size of a little kid's tricycle, picked itself up and started following excitedly behind me, like an annoying yappy little dog. I hadn't gotten far when I noticed a commotion out on the water. I took a closer look, and it was a struggling swimmer, calling for help. A couple of rescue swimmers had paddled out on their surfboards to help her, and I jumped in and helped them back to shore. When she caught her breath, the swimmer explained that she's always wanted to do an Ironman. She was a pretty strong cyclist and runner, but she never learned how to swim. If only she could swim!

Then one of the lifeguards chimed in. He was wearing a wetsuit and standing next to his surfboard, and he looked like a swimming God. He said he's been swimming since he was born, and he could run OK, but he never had a bike. If only he could learn how to ride a bike, he was sure he could complete an Ironman.

OK, in hindsight, I probably should've told them I was on my way to see the Wizard, that he was going to teach me all the secrets of the Ironman, and maybe he could help them too. And it probably would've made a better story. But I'm a triathlete. Last thing I wanted was two more competitors. The dude with the surfboard looked like he might be in my age group. So I just went on my way. They were a bunch of whiners anyway.

As I was walking along, suddenly I was besieged by a horde of angry, maniac cyclists, hurtling toward me at breakneck speed, shrieking like a pack of deranged flying monkeys. Apparently the bike leg had begun, and I was walking in the middle of the course. It was a miracle I didn't get carried away by the pack.

Finally, after a lot of searching, I tracked down the Wizard. He was on the side of the highway, fixing a flat. It was kind of anticlimactic. Wearily, he said there was no secret. He said I've had it in me all along to run a strong marathon. All I had to do was train a little harder.

Gee, thanks. Very helpful. I was hoping for something more along the lines of a magic pair of running shoes.

Unqualified Support for the Ironman

A couple years ago, a good friend of mine named Nic decided he would try to qualify for the Hawaii Ironman. It made perfect sense to him. He was going to be in Hawaii anyway, since he was getting married there, and by total coincidence the wedding just happened to be the same weekend as the race. So what the heck. Why not give it a shot?

Well, we all figured that Nic would come close, but that he wouldn't quite make it. To the altar, that is. The Ironman, we figured, was a sure thing. Nic is probably one of the more intense creatures who ever lived. He had been an elite local triathlete for about two decades, and his training regimen was legendary. So we figured if he put his mind to it, which he pretty much always did, he'd get in no problem.

It therefore came as quite a shock to us locals, who had been eating his dust for all those years, when Nic came up a couple minutes short of a qualifying spot. After it was over, I thought maybe his attempt to qualify might make a good subject for a story, so I asked him, cautiously, if there was anything amusing about his effort to get into the race that he could pass along.

When I posed the question, Nic took it, as he does most everything, very seriously. He paused for a while to give it his full consideration. And then he looked at me and said: "No, there was absolutely nothing amusing about it."

Did I mention that Nic is an extremely serious guy, a person not prone to flights of exaggeration? When he said that there was absolutely nothing amusing about his attempt to qualify for the Ironman, what he meant was that, literally, there was *absolutely nothing amusing about it*. Now bear in mind that this is a guy who had practically staged his own wedding in order to create the opportunity to do the race — a fact that most neutral observers would find, I think, meets the "amusing" threshold. That will give you an idea of how much fun it is to nearly kill yourself trying to qualify for Kona, and not quite make it.

The truth is, the deck is stacked against the Nics of the world from the beginning. There was only one qualifying race in New England, and it happened to be last qualifying race anywhere, period, and so every desperate triathlete in the known universe came out of the woodwork. Suddenly, instead of competing against all the same local folks he's been beating up on for years, now Nic's getting passed by guys named Gunter screaming "on your left" in German. With only three qualifying slots and a couple hundred people in your age group, things start getting pretty tough. This must be how American distance runners feel when they're used to being total studs at the University of Arkansas or wherever, and then they enter an international race and all of a sudden they're finishing behind entire villages of Kenyans and Ethiopians.

And then, of course, the final indignity is knowing that there is a whole batch of folks at the starting line in Kona who didn't qualify at all, but who got in through the "lottery." I wish these people all the best, but I have to say that the whole lottery concept is bizarre to me. Competing in the Ironman is hardly the kind of windfall that one normally associates with winning a lottery. It's like getting a letter in the mail from Ed McMahon that says, in giant 24-point type, "CONGRATULATIONS! YOU MAY HAVE ALREADY WON 12 HOURS OF EXCRUCIATING MISERY AND PAIN!!"

The Real Ironmen

"Honey, guess what!"

"What?"

"You know all that practicing I've been doing on the piano? All those early morning scales? All those sore, aching fingers?"

"Yeah . . ."

"Well, I got great news! I've been invited to play in a very big recital!"

"A recital! Wow, that's great, congratulations!"

"Thanks. You'll come watch, right . . . ?"

"Of course I'll come watch."

"Great! It's in Hawaii in October!"

"Hawaii!? Why do you have to go all the way to Hawaii for a piano recital? Aren't there plenty of recitals around here?"

"Well, this is a very *special* recital. But if you don't want to go, that's fine, I can go by myself . . ."

"No, no . . . Of course I'll go . . ."

"OK good. Now just so you know, it's going to be, um . . . kind of a long recital . . ."

"What do you mean long? How long?"

"Well, it depends, but probably somewhere around, oh, 11 hours, if all goes well."

"*Eleven hours*!?!"

"Yep. We're playing Beethoven's Ninth Symphony 6,000 consecutive times!"

"OK, you're joking right?"

"No honey, I'm serious. And bring your suntan lotion!"

"Suntan lotion? Why would I need suntan lotion?"

"Because the recital is outside, and it can get hot in Hawaii in October. And windy. Of course it can also rain, and this recital goes on rain or shine!"

"Oh great . . ."

"Honey! I really thought you'd be excited about this!"

"Of course I'm excited to watch you play."

"Well, that's another thing . . ."

"What?"

"You might not actually get to see me play all that much . . ."

"Why not??"

"Well, um, most of the actual recital takes place pretty far away from where the spectators are. So, for most of the time, you'll be looking at this big giant stage with lots and lots of really expensive abandoned pianos. And then every couple of hours, I'll stop by and play a couple notes."

"Gee, that sounds like great fun . . ."

"Now don't be sarcastic . . . This is very important to me."

"OK, I'm sorry. Well if it's that long, at least I'll be able to go do some sightseeing in Hawaii, or maybe some shopping.

"What?! You can't do that, I need you there to support me!"

"But you just said I'm hardly ever going to see you!"

"Yeah, but you need to be there when I come by! What if I forget, like, a critical piece of sheet music or something? I'll need you to run out to the car to grab it. You're my crew!"

"I thought you said you're playing the same piece of music 6,000 times. I would think you'd have it pretty much down pat."

"OK Captain Sarcasm, if you don't want to help that's fine, I can do it myself."

"OK don't pout, I'll be your crew . . . So Hawaii huh, that's gotta be expensive. I assume they're paying your expenses?"

"No, silly! We're lucky just to get invited! And the entry fee is only $650."

"*Entry fee*?! Are you kidding? You're going all the way to Hawaii to play in this recital and *they're* charging *you* $650?"

"Yep. Oh, there's one other thing . . ."

"What?"

"Well . . . I think I need a new piano."

"What?!?! Whats wrong with your piano?"

"There's nothing *wrong* with it, it's just not good enough for a recital like this, trust me. But don't worry, I found this awesome new piano on the Internet. And its only $3,000."

"Oh brother . . ."

"Shipping it to Hawaii might get a little pricey though."

"Please let this be a nightmare . . ."

The Enronman Triathlon

In the wake of the accounting scandals that have rocked the corporate world, I would like to propose a new type of triathlon: The Enronman. Officially, the Enronman would go in the books as an Ironman-distance triathlon. You can tell your friends you completed an Ironman-distance race. Race directors can charge Ironman-like entry fees. But behind the scenes, the race will consist of nothing more than an easy, three-mile jog, followed by beer and pizza. Hey, if corporate executives have been doing it for years, I don't see why we shouldn't go along for the ride.

I don't mean to make light of the situation on Wall Street. These corporate scandals are serious business. And they should serve as a wake-up call to all of us triathletes. Because it's only a matter of time before the lawyers and regulators get bored and turn their attention from Wall Street to the Queen K Highway. We all know that there are some, shall we say, irregularities that go on in our sport as well.

Those of you who are training for an Ironman know what I mean. As the big day approaches, don't tell me there isn't some serious double booking of workouts going on out there. It just doesn't seem possible to get in the kind of mileage that all those training charts and articles require, so, like a desperate corporate exec trying to pad his first-quarter results, you inflate the numbers a little bit here or there, figuring you'll make it up on your next long brick workout. It becomes a giant training Ponzi scheme. If you've given in to this temptation, trust me, now is the time to start tossing those training logs into the shredder. Because when race day finally arrives, the Ironman is going to be the mother of all audits, I can assure you.

Training isn't the only place where there are some shady accounting practices going on. There's going to have to be a crackdown on the reporting of race results as well. Like quarterly reports from struggling corporations, we all have a natural tendency to try to make our results look as attractive as possible. The urge is particularly strong in a race like the Ironman, where the level of competition is so high. This is why we have age groups: "I finished 19th in my age group!" sounds a heck of a lot better than, "I finished in the bottom 10 percent overall."

Sometimes, though, this urge causes us to stretch the truth a bit. I have to admit that I've been a repeat offender. I finished my first Ironman, back in 1999, in 12:31. Whenever anyone asks me how I did, I can't seem to keep from saying "Oh, right around 12 hours!" In my mind, that's close enough, but if there were a Triathlon Exchange Commission (and it's only a matter of time), I'm pretty sure they'd consider it a material misrepresentation. Like some CEOs these days, I live in constant fear that someone is going to look behind the surface and uncover the real numbers.

Then there are all those races that you don't even bother to tell anyone about. You know the ones I mean, the races where you made a bad cheeseburger-related decision the night before and where you decide, somewhere around the beginning of the bike leg, that this is just going to be a training race. Somehow, these races never seem to make it into the reports of your results for the season. They're off-balance-sheet races. In my case, I've created a fictitious general partnership in which to conceal these races. I'm sure it won't be long before the subpoenas start showing up at my doorstep. At least I'll be able to outrun the process servers.

Does the Road to Kona Have a Breakdown Lane?

I still remember, years and years ago, the first time I heard about Ironman. Like a lot of people of my generation, I saw it on *Wide World of Sports*. I was in high school at the time, and about the only thing I did to stay in shape was play basketball and make an occasional beer run.

So I can say with complete confidence that, as I watched this crazy event on TV, I'm sure I would have bet everything I owned — admittedly, at the time this was not much more than a pair of Converse high-tops and a poster of Dr. J — that I would walk on the moon before I'd compete in an event like the Ironman. I watched the race with the same kind of bemused detachment with which I would have watched other comically absurd feats of endurance and obsession, the kind you might read about in the *Guinness Book of World Records*, like pogo-sticking for 37 days straight.

Even after I survived my first tri, vividly chronicled in the first chapter of this book, and slowly started getting more involved in the sport, the Ironman never crossed my mind. Ironman was reserved for endurance freaks who were born with a different set of DNA. But then I finally got a marathon under my belt. And the next season I was talked into training for a half Ironman, and managed to survive it in reasonably decent shape. Little by little, the absurdity of the Ironman distance started fading away, to the point where all of a sudden it no longer seemed quite so preposterous. Intimidating and terrifying, yes, but not preposterous.

And so, roughly 20 years after seeing the Ironman for the first time on TV and thinking it was an outlandish freak show, I became one of the freaks and signed up for my first Ironman race. As an Ironman survivor, I thought I would take this opportunity to pass along some advice to those of you who might be about to tackle the Ironman for the first time.

The first thing I will tell you is that they are not kidding about the distance. They really do make you cover every inch of the 2.4-, 112- and 26.2-mile course. This was a bit of a disappointment to me. The distance is so absurd, I figured somewhere around the half-way point there would be a race official on the course, discretely motioning competitors toward a secret, air-conditioned chamber, where everyone is sitting around chatting and drinking beer, waiting a respectable period of time before heading off on a shortcut that would take us to a spot much further along on the course. Unfortunately, that never happened . . . although about 15 miles into the run I did have a couple of hallucinations that came close.

Since they're serious about the distance, it's probably a good idea to come somewhere in the general neighborhood of those distances during your training. Take it from me, a 60-mile bike and five-mile run is not in the general neighborhood. It can be very tempting to try to rationalize this kind of "long" workout, and your brain will play all kinds of tricks on you. "You don't want to burn yourself out!" "Wouldn't want to overtrain and risk injury!" Don't believe any of it. You've got to put in the distance. And if you do overtrain and get hurt, the good news is you'll have the perfect excuse to avoid the actual race, so it's kind of a win-win.

Another piece of advice, and this may sound counter-intuitive, is that you should refrain from speaking to anyone who knows anything about the Ironman — and preferably anyone who knows anything about the sport of triathlon — for a minimum of five months prior to the race. I don't know whether they do it on purpose, but other triathletes will almost certainly say something to cause you to have a nervous breakdown over the inadequacy of your own preparations. Maybe it will be the details of their own training regimen, which will inevitably dwarf your own pathetic workouts, or maybe it will be some horror story about a failed Ironman attempt. I remember running into a local triathlete during a training ride before my first Ironman. The race was still several months away, but this guy asked me, with a perfectly straight face, if I had started tapering yet. Of course, I did the only thing I could do in that situation — I stuck my frame pump into the spokes of his front wheel and went on my way.

The actual race-day logistics of an Ironman can also be a bit intimidating if you aren't adequately prepared. At a "normal" triathlon, you can dump your gear pretty much wherever you want when you set up your little spot in the transition area on race morning. This allows you to stop at a 24-hour convenience store on the way to the race in the morning, purchase all your critical last-minute supplies (for me, usually Ibuprofen and Rolaids), and generally deal with everything in a completely frenzied, last-minute panic. This suits my lifestyle perfectly.

Ironman requires an entirely different set of organizational skills. You have to pack your transition bags and hang them in the proper spots in the transition area the day before the race. This was a radical concept for me. For some reason, it is much more stressful to pack those bags the day before. The problem is that there is just way too much time to think about what to put in there, and way too much time afterwards to think about what you forgot. I unpacked and repacked those bags so many times that when I finally got to the transition area during the race, I couldn't even remember what I'd put in there. It felt like the day after Halloween, when you got to dump out the contents of your trick-or-treat bag. I felt like turning to the guy next to me in the transition area and asking him what he got.

Anyway, I hope these reflections are helpful to all you first-timers out there, and I hope you take them to heart as you prepare for what will be one of the most challenging, rewarding and absurd experiences of your life. And, most of all, I hope that you've already started tapering.

Awards Presentation

Like staging a triathlon, putting this book together wouldn't have been possible without help from a ton of people. Properly thanking everyone is about as realistic as running the perfect race, but, like a delusional age-grouper who goes out there every weekend thinking it's all finally gonna come together, I'm going to give it a shot. First, I'd like to thank the folks at *Inside Triathlon* who, "back in the day," took a chance on me and my silly triathlon column and gave me my first opportunity to see my writing in print. I had a number of great editors over the years including Chris Newbound, Anne Stein, and Cameron Elford. Thanks to Cassie Lee-Trettel at Competitor Group, who helped me search old archives of *Inside Triathlon* to track down some missing columns. Much gratitude as well to all of the great people at FriesenPress who helped me see this project through to conclusion, including Lynn Wohlgemuth, Eric Anderson and Amanda Eyolfson. Thanks to all of the people who graciously agreed to review drafts of this book, including most notably my parents, Nathan and Eva Dodell, Ulandt Kim and Dan Margolies. A grudging thank you to all of my training and racing partners over the decades, people like Nic Scibelli, Ulandt Kim, Bill Nuzzo, Scott Phillips, Jay Courant and many others, all of whom are far better athletes than me, but who nevertheless let me tag along and never made too much fun of me (at least not to my face). And finally, I'd like to thank all the race directors and volunteers who, for reasons I will never quite understand, work tirelessly week after week, year after year to make sure we'll have an opportunity to get up at a stupidly early hour every weekend and try to kill ourselves!

About the Author

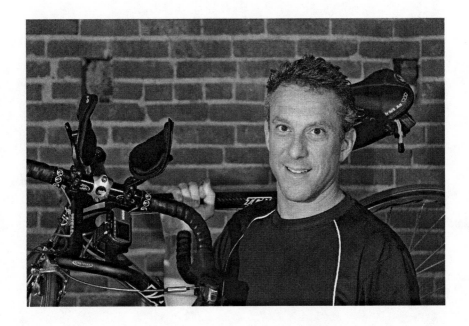

Photograph by Dave Kaup Photography

Leib Dodell is an attorney, writer and extremely amateur triathlete (some would say extremely amateur attorney and writer as well). For a dozen years, Leib wrote a column called "The Lighter Side" in *Inside Triathlon* magazine, focusing on the trials and tribulations of the average triathlete (as if there were such a thing). He currently lives in Kansas City, MO with his dog Bear, where he (Leib) runs a specialty underwriting agency providing professional liability insurance to publishers, authors, websites, advertisers and other media and technology companies. This is his first book.

CPSIA information can be obtained at www.ICGtesting.com
Printed in the USA
LVOW060047151011

250640LV00004B/1/P